Health Promotion
Practice

Health Promotion Practice

Building Empowered Communities

Glenn Laverack

Open University Press

Open University Press
McGraw-Hill Education
McGraw-Hill House
Shoppenhangers Road
Maidenhead
Berkshire
England
SL6 2QL

email: enquiries@openup.co.uk
world wide web: www.openup.co.uk

and Two Penn Plaza, New York, NY 10121–2289, USA

First published 2007

A catalogue record of this book is available from the British Library

ISBN– 10: 0335 220 576 (pb)   0335 220 584 (hb)
ISBN– 13: 978 0 335 220 571 (pb)   978 0 335 220 588 (hb)

Library of Congress Cataloguing-in-Publication Data
CIP data applied for

Typeset by YHT Ltd, London
Printed by Printed in Poland by OZ Graf. S. A.
www.polskabook.pl

The *McGraw-Hill* Companies

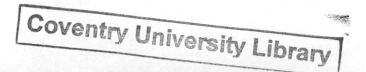

Contents

Tables, Figures and Boxes

Tables

Figures

Boxes

Preface

I grew up in a single-parent family at the bottom of the social and economic gradient and draw on my personal experiences in Chapter 3. My work in public health and health promotion over the past 25 years has always been with those who have to suffer the consequences of poverty and inequality. Throughout my life I have observed the powerlessness of others or have myself been directly affected by those who have power over my health and its determinants. This will continue to motivate me to write about and to work with people who struggle to gain power.

The idea for this book began when I was working on a school health promotion programme in southern India. It was typically top-down with control over decisions and resources taken by an outside agent that also designed, implemented and evaluated the programme. This created an imbalance in power and a continual struggle for control between the Indian authorities and the outside agent. The parties involved were bound by the bureaucratic procedures imposed by the conditions of funding, lines of management and the 'milestones' imposed for meeting outcomes. The outside agent would not relinquish control because it was concerned with the effectiveness (costs and targets met) and accountability of the programme. This situation increasingly frustrated the Indian counterparts, who as the recipients felt that they already had the necessary skills and competencies to implement the programme.

At the time I strongly believed that there had to be a practical solution to reconcile these differences and my opportunity came when I went to Australia to begin my research on empowerment. My aim was to understand how programmes could be an empowering experience for the intended beneficiaries by strengthening their capacity. To achieve this I would have to tread a fine line between theory (academic excellence) and practice (pragmatism), to produce something that was rigorous and useful to the stakeholders of health promotion programmes. I began by unpacking the concept of community empowerment into its individual components. This involved a rigorous process of review and led to the categorization of what I termed the 'empowerment domains', discussed in Chapter 5.

I now had a theoretically and empirically 'rich' basis for the development of an approach to empower communities and carried out its field-testing in Fiji. This worked well and I was also able to develop the idea of 'parallel tracking' to accommodate empowerment approaches into top-down programming. This involves the strengthening of the links between the 'health promotion track' and the 'empowerment track' of the programme and provides a broader framework in which to situate the tool. I discuss this in Chapter 4. The approaches discussed in this book are now being adapted and applied in Asia, North America, the Pacific and Africa and I refer to some of these experiences in Chapters 7 and 8.

It is hoped that the book will inspire practitioners to work in more empowering ways in health promotion and to contemplate how they can influence the way others gain power.

Glenn Laverack, Auckland, New Zealand

Acknowledgements

I would like to acknowledge the many people with whom I have had the privilege of working during the course of writing this book.

In particular I would like to thank Dr Peter Adams, Dr Chris Bullen, Dr Susan Rifkin, Dr Kirsten Havemann, Dr Janine Wiles and Dr Pat Neuwelt. In Canada, Georgia Bell-Woodard, Ronald Labonte, Karen Chad and Lori Littlejohns and the staff of the SLLP project in Kyrgyzstan.

I owe much thanks to my family, Elizabeth, Ben, Holly and Rebecca, for their continued love and to my mother, Barbara, who provided the motivation for writing this book.

Introduction: an overview of the book

This book is the third in a series of publications that focus on power and empowerment in professional practice. The first two books, *Health Promotion: Power and Empowerment* (Laverack 2004) and *Public Health: Power, Empowerment and Professional Practice* (Laverack 2005) were written to provide a theoretical understanding of the subject area. This book goes further by providing a special focus on communities and is illustrated throughout with useful case study experiences. The book is written for health promotion students and practitioners who want to learn more about practical approaches that they can use to build empowered communities.

The book has three main purposes:

1   Chapters 1 to 3 provide the reader with an understanding of the key concepts used in the book and the link to improved health outcomes in the context of health promotion programmes.
2   Chapters 4 to 6 provide the reader with an understanding of practical approaches that can be used in health promotion programming to build and evaluate empowered communities.
3   Chapters 7 to 9 provide the reader with case study examples of how communities can be empowered in practice and a conclusion of the main issues discussed in the book.

Chapter 1 introduces the reader to the key concepts used in the book, including health promotion, power and empowerment, and how they are used to develop an empowering professional practice.

Chapter 2 defines and discusses, in a practical sense, the concepts of community, civil society and community-based interaction. This chapter clarifies the overlap between the key community-based concepts such as community participation, community development and community capacity and situates them in relation to community empowerment. The complexity of the difference between these and other concepts is explained, for the first time, as a ladder of community based interaction.

Chapter 3 begins with an interpretation of the different meanings of health and then provides a discussion of the link between empowerment and improved health outcomes. The chapter also examines the link between the determinants of health and empowerment and the relevance of this to health promotion practice.

Chapter 4 provides a discussion of the tensions that exist in health promotion between bottom-up and top-down styles of programming. Readers are introduced to a methodology for accommodating these two styles together within the same programme through the use of 'parallel tracking'. The application of this approach is explained by using a practical case study example of chronic disease prevention in Polynesian people in New Zealand.

Chapter 5 provides a detailed description of the nine 'domains' of community empowerment and uses case study examples to illustrate their importance to health promotion. The chapter describes a step-by-step approach for building empowered communities within health promotion programming including setting a baseline, strategic planning, implementing a strategic approach and evaluation.

Chapter 6 discusses the importance of, and provides the means to, evaluate community empowerment. It discusses the key areas of consideration when designing an evaluation methodology and offers a practical method of visual representation using the spidergram configuration. Examples of the practical use of the spidergram are given to show how this approach can be used to share information between stakeholders.

Chapter 7 provides two case study examples of how, within an *issue-based approach*, to build empowered communities by using the nine domains discussed in Chapter 5. The examples consider improving health outcomes and community capacity in Canada, and improving housing standards in an inner-city area in England.

Chapter 8 provides two case study examples of how, in a *community-based approach*, to build empowered communities by using the nine 'domains' discussed in Chapter 5. The case studies consider improving health and hygiene in a remote community in Northern Australia, and improving livelihoods in rural communities in Kyrgyzstan.

The final chapter brings together the central themes of the book, discusses the main lessons learnt from empowerment approaches and examines three different contexts in which health promoters can build empowered communities: social, structural and radical.

1 Health promotion practice

Health promotion in context

While there is no singularly accepted definition of health promotion, the term is generally regarded as a multi-faceted process involving individuals, 'interest' groups and communities. The operational purpose of health promotion is to enable people to increase control over, and to improve, their health and its determinants. This is embodied in the *Ottawa Charter for Health Promotion* (WHO 1986) and the *Bangkok Charter for Health Promotion in a Globalized World* (WHO 2005):

The *Ottawa Charter* states:

> Health promotion is the process of enabling people to increase control over, and to improve, their health. To reach a state of complete physical, mental and social well-being, an individual or group must be able to identify and to realize aspirations, to satisfy needs and to change or cope with the environment. Health is, therefore, seen as a resource for everyday life, not the objective of living. Health is a positive concept emphasizing social and personal resources, as well as physical capacities. Therefore, health promotion is not just the responsibility of the health sector, but goes beyond healthy lifestyles to well-being.
>
> (WHO 1986: 1)

The *Bangkok Charter* states:

> The United Nations recognizes that the enjoyment of the highest attainable standard of health is one of the fundamental rights of everyday human being without discrimination. Health promotion is based on this critical human right and offers a positive and inclusive concept of health as a determinant of the quality of life and encompassing mental and spiritual well-being. Health promotion is the process of enabling people to increase control over their health and its determinants, and thereby improve their health. It is a core function of public health and contributes to the work of tackling communicable and non-communicable diseases and other threats to health.
>
> (WHO 2005: 1)

In the period between the publication of the *Ottawa Charter* in 1986 and the *Bangkok Charter* in 2005, the core theme in health promotion remained unchanged: enabling people to increase control over their lives and health. This is the process of empowerment in which the practitioner acts as a facilitator to assist the individuals, groups and communities with whom they work to gain more power. Power is the level of control that their clients have over access to resources, choices and decisions. The implications of power and empowerment to health promotion practice are central to this book.

Unlike the *Ottawa Charter*, the *Bangkok Charter* does not provide a framework that health promotion practitioners can use to directly help to empower their clients. The *Bangkok Charter* is intended for a different audience: governments and politicians at all levels, the private sector, international organizations as well as civil society and the public health community. The four commitments of the *Bangkok Charter* are to make the promotion of health central to the global development agenda and a core responsibility for all of government, to make health promotion a key focus for communities and civil society and a requirement for good corporate practice. These commitments require strong intergovernmental and corporate agreements and action. Unfortunately, the *Bangkok Charter* does not presently provide a clear role for practitioners or a 'plan of action' indicating who, how and when the commitments will be achieved. The experience of the *Ottawa Charter* has shown that social and political change (empowerment) has a better chance of success when it is backed by a 'movement' of professionals and civil society.

Health promotion is most often delivered as a planned set of activities within the design of an intervention, a project or a programme, and controlled by government departments, agencies or government-funded non-governmental organizations (NGOs). In this book I have used the term 'programme' to refer to all these circumstances. Within a programme context there is always some power relationship between different people, primarily between practitioners and their clients. Practitioners are employed to deliver information, resources and services and are often seen as an outside agent to the people who benefit and who are their clients. Many of these people call themselves 'health promotion practitioners' or 'public health practitioners' while many more who look to the idea of health promotion occupy roles such as nurses, environmental health officers, housing officers and doctors. In this book I refer to all these people as 'practitioners'. Their 'clients' cover the range of people with whom they work, including women, adolescents, men and other professional groups (Laverack 2005).

Practitioners are expected to display a specialization of knowledge, technical competence, social responsibility and service to their clients. Their level of professionalism is attained through education, training, professional codes of practice and core competencies. Core competencies are a combination of attributes that enable an individual to perform a set of tasks to an appropriate standard. Core competencies for health promotion not only include practical knowledge and skills but also the values and principles that shape professional practice. Core competencies also provide a set of standards by which the workforce can determine what 'professional' practice is and can be used to set parameters for staff development, recruitment and performance standards.

However, for some practitioners health promotion is only a part of their daily work – for example, a nurse who undertakes a mix of clinical practice and health education. Different professional groups have developed their own sets of generic competencies. These provide the minimum entry level of competence to meet a professional standard – for example, to deliver essential nursing services. Practitioners who are not solely involved in health promotion have a responsibility to select which specialist competencies they feel are most relevant to their work.

Box 1.1 provides a list of competencies that although not exhaustive are fundamental in allowing health promotion practitioners to grow and to develop as professionals.

Box 1.1   Core competencies for health promotion programming

1 Programme design, management, implementation and evaluation
The ability to plan effective health promotion programmes, including the management of resources and personnel. This involves an understanding of programme cycles, budgeting, and the planning and evaluation of bottom-up approaches in top down programming.

2 The planning and delivery of effective communication strategies
Communication strategies are an integral part of many health promotion programmes to increase knowledge levels and to raise awareness. A high level of competence is needed for the development of programmes that target individuals, groups and communities, including one-to-one communication, the design of print materials and the use of the mass media.

3 Facilitating skills
Training (e.g. for skills development, usually within a workshop setting) is a key part of many health promotion programmes. Good facilitation skills are essential for health promoters and are an important part of programme design.

4 Research skills
Health promotion programme design and evaluation is based on sound research including the use of participatory techniques, qualitative and quantitative methods and systematic reviews.

5 Community capacity-building skills

Community empowerment is central to health promotion. This is a process of capacity-building and health promoters must be competent in a range of strategies that they can use to help individuals, groups and communities to gain more power.

6 Ability to influence policy and practice

Health promoters have the opportunity to influence policy and practice in their everyday work, for example, through technical advisory groups and through helping communities to mobilize and organize themselves towards gaining power. Health promoters must develop competence in the use of strategies to influence policy, developing partnerships and sound working relationships.

Box 1.2 provides a new definition of health promotion to describe it as both a set of principles and as a practice within the context of these core competencies.

Box 1.2   A new definition of health promotion

Health promotion is a set of principles (e.g. equity, compassion) centred around the concept of empowerment to enable people to take more control over the de-terminants of their lives and health. Health promotion practice encompasses a range of communication, capacity-building and politically orientated approaches set within a programme context. Health promotion practitioners use these ap-proaches to help their clients (individuals, groups, organizations and communities) to gain more power (control) over decisions and resources regarding their health.

As already stated, the purpose of health promotion practice is to enable others to gain more control over their health and its determinants. When we think of health promotion practice in these terms it is clear that the purpose of everything we do as practitioners is to help our clients, the individuals, groups and communities with whom we work, to gain more power. For example, many activities in health promotion directly relate to power:

- Health communication and health education strategies are used to increase knowledge levels and raise awareness so that clients can make informed choices about the decisions regarding their lives and health. The control over decision-making, of which access to accurate information is an important element, is one form of power-over (discussed later in this chapter).
- Training, role play, work experience and counselling are examples of how practitioners help their clients to develop the necessary skills to take more control over the situations in their lives, including their health.

- Community development, community organization, community participation and community capacity-building are fundamentally forms of social organization and collective action aimed at redressing inequalities in the distribution of power. Health promoters use these approaches to increase the assets and attributes which individuals in a community are able to draw upon in order to take control of their lives.

Plainly put, the role of health promotion practitioners is to enable their clients to gain control over the determinants of their health. A practical way in which health promoters can do this is through the redistribution of power, a central theme of this book.

Health promotion and public health

The *Bangkok Charter* positions health promotion as 'a core function of public health [that] contributes to the work of tackling communicable and non-communicable diseases and other threats to health' (WHO 2005: 1). In a programming context, public health and health promotion exist as equal partners and provide practitioners with conceptual models, strategic approaches and professional legitimacy.

Public health, like health promotion, is a contested term given the wide range of competing perspectives, priorities and services that it claims to deliver. It is an approach that aims to promote health, prevent disease, treat illness, care for the infirm and provide health services. Such a broad range of goals also means that the term 'public health' is used to cover a number of specialist areas including nursing and health promotion. Public health involves working with individuals, groups and 'communities', incorporates methods that connect collective action to the broader aims of political influence and competes for limited resources and control over decisions. Power and empowerment are therefore core concepts to a public health practice that seeks to redress inequalities in health and to change the determinants of health through community-based interaction.

Health promotion and public health are similar in that they:

- address the determinants of health by working towards changing inequalities in society, for example, providing equality of access to information about lifestyle issues such as smoking and physical inactivity;
- enable their clients to gain more power through a process of empowerment involving specific strategies to help individuals, groups and communities to take control of their lives and health;
- employ communication approaches to raise awareness and increase

knowledge levels to improve the lives and health of their clients, including the mass media, printed materials, face-to-face communication, social marketing and information, education and communication.

Box 1.3 provides a series of statements that give examples of the wide range of activities that can be covered by public health and health promotion practitioners. Answering 'yes' would indicate a broad view of what is classified as health promotion. Answering 'no' would indicate a narrow view of what health promotion is, for example, that some activities are health education without considering this within a wider definition. When completing this exercise, either as an individual or in a group setting, ask yourself what are the reasons for selecting 'yes' or 'no'? What are the criteria you have used in making this selection?

Box 1.3 What is health promotion?

Consider each of the following statements, and decide whether you think each activity is or is not health promotion:

Yes / No

Using the mass media to inform people of healthy practices.

Assisting a 'community' to prepare a petition against the site for an electrical pylon.

Explaining to clients how to carry out the advice of a doctor.

In an advisory committee you support the use of 'speed bumps' outside schools.

Developing leaflets on home safety for distribution to the elderly.

Running exercise classes for women in ethnic groups.

Raising awareness about how powerlessness affects health.

Providing skills training on the proper use of condoms to youth groups.

Counselling someone on how to cope with domestic violence.

(Adapted from Ewles and Simnett 2003: 27)

Health promotion and health education

Practitioners are sometimes confused by the differences between the terms health promotion and health education. This is because in practice they both employ similar methods to inform people and to develop individual skills. The debate about the overlap between health promotion and health education began in the 1980s when the range of activities involved in promoting better health widened to overcome the narrow focus on lifestyle and behaviour approaches. These activities involved more than just giving information and aimed for strategies that achieved political action and social mobilization.

Some authors (e.g. Tones *et al.* 2001) have suggested that health education and health promotion have a symbiotic relationship. Health education provides the agenda-setting and critical consciousness-raising in health promotion programmes. Without the inclusion of education strategies, health promotion programmes would be little more than manipulative processes of social coercion and community control. But, whereas health education is aimed at informing people to influence their future decision-making, health promotion aims at complementary social and political actions. These include lobbying and community development that facilitate political changes in people's social, workplace and community environments to enhance health (Green and Kreuter 1991). Thus, health education around obesity issues might include school-based awareness programmes or exercise classes. Health promotion around obesity extends to legislation on food advertising and restricting access to unhealthy products in school shops. The most practical way forward is to view health promotion as encompassing health education as a range of educational activities.

Next is an interpretation of the concepts of power and empowerment in health promotion practice: power-over; power from within and power-with. These concepts are discussed in detail elsewhere (Laverack 2004, 2005) and here an overview is provided of why these concepts are important to the work of health promotion practitioners.

Power and powerlessness

Power-over

The most common western interpretation of power used in health promotion practice is in the form of one person or group having control over others; the resources or decisions that influence their lives and health. This is power-over. In the context of power-over the resources which a practitioner may bring to bear on their client in order to change their beliefs, attitudes and behaviours have been identified as six bases of *social power-over* (Raven and Litman-Adizes

1986). This is the relationship between people in which a more 'powerful person' or group has power over others through coercion, reward, legitimacy, expertise, reference and information.

In *coercive power*, the practitioner may bring about negative consequences or punishment for a person if they do not comply, for example by scolding a mother for not breastfeeding their child.

In *reward power*, the practitioner may bring about positive consequences for the person upon compliance, for example by praising a mother for breastfeeding her child and keeping the child clean.

Legitimate power stems from the person accepting a social role relationship with the practitioner, a structural relationship which grants them the right to prescribe behaviour for the person, while the person accepts an obligation to comply with the requests of the practitioner. For example, the person accepts the legitimate professional position of a nurse and listens to and carries out her advice.

Expert power stems from the person attributing superior knowledge and ability to the practitioner, for example the term 'doctor knows best' illustrates the expert power relationship between the patient and doctor.

Referent power stems from an identification of the person with the practitioner, a feeling of communality, similarity and mutual interest. The person then gets some satisfaction from believing and complying in a manner consistent with the beliefs, attitudes and behaviours of the practitioner.

Informational power is based on the explicit information communicated to the person from the practitioner, a persuasive communication that will convince them that the recommended behaviour is indeed in their best interests, for example advice on appropriate forms of family planning to assist child spacing. Informational power is the form commonly used in health education.

The concept of power-over can also be viewed as both a limited, finite entity (zero sum) and as an expanding, infinite entity (non-zero sum). Zero sum power exists when one can only possess X amount of power to the extent that someone else has the absence of an equivalent amount. It is therefore a 'win/lose' situation. My power over you, plus your absence of that power, equals zero (thus the term 'zero sum'). I win and you lose. For you to gain power, you must seize it from me. If you can, you win and I lose. Power is used as leverage to raise the position of one person or group, while simultaneously lowering it for another person or group. However, at any one time there will be only so much leverage (wealth, control, resources etc.) possessed within a society. The role of the practitioner is to enable their clients to gain more control of resources or decision-making that influence their health and lives, over and in competition with other individuals and groups.

Non-zero sum power is regarded not as fixed and finite, but as infinite and expanding and offers a 'win/win' situation since it is based on the idea that if any one person or group gains, everyone else also gains. Non-zero sum power takes the form of building equitable working relationships based on respect, generosity, service to others, a free flow of information and the commitment to the ethics of caring and justice. The role of the practitioner is to use these attributes to create a partnership with their clients and to transfer power by encouraging others to gain the skills necessary to access resources and information (Laverack 2004).

To enable their clients to gain power from others, practitioners must firstly identify their own power bases before they can be shared with others. To do this, practitioners must understand both how to use their own power bases to help themselves into a position of more control and how to help others to gain power. Practitioners generally do have more power or a stronger power base than their clients, for example as a consequence of their education and professional training, high incomes, expert status, a higher position on the social gradient, access to information and resources, influence over decision-makers, familiarity with systems of bureaucracy and control over budgets. This raises an ethical dilemma: which groups, at the expense of others, should get priority of the limited resources and assistance from the practitioner? What criteria should be used to select one group or community in preference to another?

In everyday life, to exercise choice is the simplest form of power-over. This may involve the trivial health choice of buying different brands of health care products such as toothpaste or the more critical choices about whether or not to stop smoking. Power-over is resource dependent and is viewed as being 'capacity' reliant on some type of material product. This essentially ignores that power must also be a property of social relations including the relationship one has with oneself (Clegg 1989).

To the extent that our personal choices also constrain those of others, power then becomes an exercise of control. Our ability to control decisions can condition and constrain the ability of other people to exercise control or choice – for example, a mother who smokes while pregnant or who chooses to feed her children unhealthy food. People therefore have control (power)-over themselves, over others and are also acted upon (constrained, influenced) by those that have control over them.

To better understand how power can be exercised in both a positive manner and a negative manner, it is helpful for practitioners to consider two other variations: power from within and 'power-with'.

Power from within

Power from within can be described as a personal power or some inner sense of self-knowledge, self-discipline and strength (Labonte 1996). Power from within is also known as individual, personal or psychological power, the means of gaining (a sense of) control over one's life (Rissel 1994). The goal of is to increase feelings of personal value and a sense of individual control. Individual control is in part a consequence of the position of people in structural and social hierarchies and has been shown to have an influence on their health. Richard Wilkinson (1996: 182) found that people who experience low income, less control in their lives and at work and who had a poor education are more likely to experience ill health. It seems that the higher one's position in the workplace or society, and the higher one's control, wealth and status, the better one's health. The findings from the workplace studies were also thought to have domestic equivalents in terms of control over money. Problems of employment or housing insecurity are a symptom of poor income, and the more money a person has the greater choice and control they have to overcome such problems. What this means is that, for example, income distribution is an important determinant of the power from within of individuals. However, a central premise of power from within is that individuals can become more powerful without gaining power over material resources such as money, social status and authority. Their inner sense of strength comes from the knowledge of their own ability to cope with and address the determinants of their health. The concept of power from within is also connected to a person's state of mental health as a: 'state of well-being in which the individual realizes his or her own abilities, can cope with the normal stresses of life, can work productively and fruitfully, and is able to make a contribution to his or her community' (WHO 2001: 1). In this positive sense, which is more than the absence of mental illness, it is the basis for mental health promotion. Like physical and social health it is also a prerequisite for individuals to participate and function in communities toward capacity-building and empowerment.

Power-with

Power-with describes a different set of social relationships, in which power-over is deliberately used to increase the power from within of another person, for example, the client, rather than to dominate them. Power-over transforms to power-with only when the less powerful person in the relationship has accrued enough power from within to exercise their own choices in regard to their health and lives. The person with the power-over (the practitioner) chooses not to exert control, but to suggest and to begin a discussion that will increase the other's (the client) sense of power from within. The practitioner offers advice to their client in the identification and resolution of problems to help develop their power from within, their abilities and inner strengths. Box 1.4 provides an example of the delicate balance in the transformative use of power-over.

Powerlessness

Powerlessness, or the absence of power, whether imagined or real, is an individual concept with the expectancy that the behaviour of a person cannot determine the outcomes they seek. It combines an attitude of self-blame, a sense of generalized distrust, a feeling of alienation from resources for social influence, an experience of disenfranchisement and economic vulnerability, and a sense of hopelessness in gaining social and political influence (Kieffer 1984). Individuals internalize their objective or external powerlessness, create a potent psychological barrier to empowering action and do not even engage in activities that meet their real needs. They begin to accept aspects of their world that are self-destructive to their own health and well-being, thinking that these are unalterable features of what they take to be 'reality' (Lerner 1986).

Box 1.4   The transformative use of power-over

The traditional doctor and patient relationship is fundamentally unequal and all competence and expertise is considered to belong to one party, the doctor. The patient voluntarily surrenders to the unspoken claim of medical (expert) power. The doctor has control over the knowledge even though that knowledge concerns the patient's own body. The attributes of health are viewed as an individual 'case' and the diagnosis is made on the basis of the medical model (the presence or absence of disease or illness) which serves to protect the legitimate and expert bases of power held by the doctor. However, in the health system the power-over relationship does not stop at diagnosis because the doctor also often controls the admission and discharge, choice of treatment, referral and care of their patient (Laverack 2005: 31).

The challenge is to strengthen individuals' power from within, partly by helping them to identify their own sources of power-over. However, some practitioners themselves feel in a position of powerlessness because of the power that others, such as their managers, have over them in a work setting. This can reduce their confidence to help others. Box 1.5 provides a simple exercise that can be used to help practitioners to begin to think critically, and discuss and support one another in regard to their own positions of powerlessness in a work setting.

Professional practice and empowerment

The transformative use of power by practitioners is the link between professional practice and empowerment. Empowerment is the means to attaining power and in the broadest sense is seen as a process by which people work together to increase control over events that influence their lives. Empowerment cannot be given but must come from within individuals and the groups that they form. In health promotion programming, those that have power or have access to it, such as practitioners, and those who want it, such as their clients, must work together to create the conditions necessary to make empowerment possible.

Box 1.5 Examining positions of powerlessness

This exercise allows the practitioner to begin to think critically. The exercise can be carried out in small groups or on an individual basis with workshop participants.

1   The participants are asked to produce a short written description of themselves in a position where the director of the health unit (or another person in authority) has power over them in their work setting.

2   The participants are then asked:

- How do you feel in this situation?
- What is the basis for your sense of powerlessness?
- How can you change the situation to make yourselves feel more comfortable?
- What simple strategies could you apply to empower yourself?

3   The participants are encouraged to discuss their answers with the whole group. The facilitator can write the main points and strategies on a board so that all the participants can see the outcome of the discussion.

Empowerment operates at three different levels: individual, organizational and community. Community empowerment is a synergistic interaction between individual empowerment, organizational empowerment and broader social and political actions. It is a dynamic process involving continual shifts in individual power (power from within) and changes in power-over relations between different social groups and decision-makers in civil society. From a practice perspective it is useful to consider community empowerment as a process along a five-point continuum representing progressively more organized and broadly-based forms of social and collective action. The continuum comprises the following elements (see Figure 1.1): Personal action; the development of small mutual groups; community organizations; partnerships; and social and political action (Laverack 1999: 92).

The continuum explains how collective action can potentially be maximized as people progress from individual to community empowerment. The continuum articulates the various levels of empowerment from personal to organizational and through collective (community) action. Each point on the continuum can be viewed as a progression toward the goals of community empowerment: social and political action and change. If not achieved the

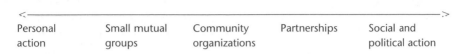

Figure 1.1   Community empowerment as a continuum
Source: Laverack (1999: 92)

community reaches stasis or can even move back to the preceding point on the continuum.

There are limitations to the concept of a continuum of community empowerment, because it offers a simple, linear interpretation of what is actually a dynamic and complex concept. The groups and organizations that arise in the process of community empowerment have their own dynamics. They may flourish for a time and then fade away for reasons as much to do with changes in the people and community as with a lack of broader political or financial support.

In this book I argue that practitioners can, and often do, play an important role in facilitating change in their clients, especially through working with groups and communities. Small mutual groups are the point at which collective action can develop further into more substantive community-based organizations. Practitioners can take a lead in the process and help groups to gain the opportunities, skills and capacities necessary to progress toward community empowerment. The practitioner must therefore be flexible in their approach to working with clients whose abilities and competencies will vary and may have to be developed. Practitioners, who are in a position of relative power, work to help their clients, who are in a relatively powerless position, to gain more control. Examples of this are the delegation of control over resources, skills development, education and advisory services, using professional influence to legitimize community concerns and lobbying for statutory change. If the practitioner is unable to achieve this progression, the group can become stagnant and develop an introspective focus on their immediate problems without developing further.

The role of the practitioner is as an 'enabler' to gain the trust of, and establish common ground with, their clients. Practitioners must also work with other professionals and agencies, both public and private, and in many other sectors, such as education, housing and social services, if they are to develop effective empowerment strategies (Laverack 2005). While practitioners cannot be expected to have an influence on transforming power relationships across all sectors and at all levels of their everyday work, they do have an important role. In practice, an empowering approach to health promotion involves helping the groups and communities in which people participate to gain power. It also means helping individuals to increase their control over the decisions which influence their lives and their participation in groups and organizations that share their concerns. Participation in 'communities of interest' is often the first step for many people towards collective action and towards using empowerment to exert a positive influence on their lives and health.

Before starting an empowering approach it is important that the practitioner is clear about their purpose and is familiar with the social, structural, political and other conditions that may influence the community. This would include, if available, a review of the epidemiological and demographic information or the collection of data using a combination of qualitative and quantitative methods. It is also important that the practitioner has identified the local meaning of key concepts such as power and empowerment. These procedures are discussed elsewhere (Laverack 1998, 2005).

Chapter 2 discusses the concepts of community and civil society and explains why the different levels of community-based interaction are so important to community empowerment and health promotion.

2 Communities and community-based interaction

This chapter addresses the reasons why some communities are more capable of accessing resources, of influencing decision-makers, are better organized and better able to mobilize themselves. It also discusses how community-based concepts relate to one another and the differences that exist between them. By using the analogy of the rungs of a ladder, it provides clarity in terms of this complex and dynamic issue.

What is a community?

It is important for practitioners to think beyond the customary view of a community as a place where people live, for example, a neighbourhood, because these are often just an aggregate of non-connected people. Communities have both social and geographic characteristics. In practice, geographic communities consist of heterogeneous individuals with dynamic social relations who may organize into groups to take action towards achieving shared goals. As a working 'rule of thumb', a community will have the following characteristics:

- a spatial dimension, that is, a place or locale;
- non-spatial dimensions (interests, issues, identities) that involve people who otherwise make up heterogeneous and disparate groups;
- social interactions that are dynamic and bind people into relationships;
- the identification of shared needs and concerns (Laverack 2004: 46).

Within the geographic or spatial dimensions of 'community', multiple non-spatial communities exist and individuals may belong to several different 'interest' groups at the same time. Interest groups exist as a legitimate means by which individuals can find a 'voice' and are able to participate in a more formal way to achieve their goals. Interest groups can be organized around a variety of issues such as social activities or the need to address a local concern, for example, the repair of a community centre. The diversity of individuals and groups within a geographic community can create problems with regard to the selection of representation by its members (Zakus and

Lysack 1998). Practitioners need to identify the 'legitimate' representatives of a community to avoid the establishment of a dominant minority that dictates community issues. Practitioners need to carefully consider if the representatives of a community are in fact supported by its members and that they are not simply acting out of self-interest. In these circumstances, a position of power-over is reached by a minority who can then direct programme activities based on their own concerns and not on those of the majority of community members.

The key role of the practitioner is to provide technical assistance and resources at the request of the community. Within an empowering approach the practitioner does not direct the community in how it should identify its representatives. The community must decide who should and who should not be their representatives. The role of the practitioner is to help all groups within the community to have a representative and to ensure that they have an equal opportunity to express their opinions.

What is civil society?

The concept of civil society includes people in both their social and professional contexts who share a common set of interests or concerns. However, it is much broader than the concept of a 'community of interest', as noted here in a definition by the London School of Economics (2006: 1):

> Civil society refers to the arena of un-coerced collective action around shared interests, purposes and values. In theory, its institutional forms are distinct from those of the state, family and market, though in practice, the boundaries between state, civil society, family and market are often complex, blurred and negotiated. Civil society commonly embraces a diversity of spaces, actors and institutional forms, varying in their degree of formality, autonomy and power. Civil societies are often populated by organisations such as registered charities, development non-governmental organisations, community groups, women's organisations, faith-based organisations, professional associations, trade unions, self-help groups, social movements, business associations, coalitions and advocacy groups.

Civil society organizations (CSOs) are also more inclusive than more traditional NGOs. They represent the totality of voluntary civic and social organizations or institutions which form the basis of a functioning society as opposed to the power-over structures of a state system. Whether all of the parties included in the above definition are a part of civil society is debatable but such a society does involve those institutions that are opposed to the state and have values of community empowerment and emancipation.

Community empowerment refers to the broad range of 'communities of interest' (social, professional, faith based etc.) that make up civil society and that are engaged in bringing about social and political change. They are discreet and organized collections of people in groups, organizations, institutions and communities situated in civil society. Their members share the same interests and have the same needs. Empowerment is the process by which the members collectively gain more control over the decisions and resources that influence their lives. Community empowerment builds from the individual to the group to a wider collective of people involved in bringing about social and political change in their favour.

What are community-based concepts?

Community-based concepts largely increase the assets and attributes that a community is able to draw upon in order to improve the lives and health of its members. Essentially, they share the same characteristics and are forms of social organization and mobilization seeking to address the inequalities in life. Over the past 30 years there has been a growth in the use of community-based concepts but with little attempt to clarify how they interact with one another or the differences that exist between them. This is because they have evolved in an ad hoc manner, sometimes to meet immediate needs and sometimes through a more thoughtful process of interpretation, usually by practitioners and academics. At a practical level there is a real need to show how these concepts can be used to enable practitioners to better interact with communities and to plan and implement health promotion programmes.

Key community-based concepts that overlap with community empowerment and that are commonly referred to in the health promotion literature include community participation (Rifkin 1990), community capacity-building (Goodman *et al.* 1998) and community development (Labonte 1998). These four concepts fundamentally share the same purpose of redressing inequalities in the distribution of power. However, these four concepts also have distinct differences and Table 2.1 provides an interpretation of how community participation, community development and community capacity relate to community empowerment.

Community-based concepts are comprised of two key characteristics: firstly, a 'community' (discussed earlier in this chapter); and secondly, the ability of its members in terms of collective social and organizational interaction. Next is an explanation of how community-based concepts interact, including the distinction between those that are concerned with participation and those that are action-orientated. Both participation and action can

Table 2.1   Three community-based concepts and their relationship to empowerment

Community empowerment is a process by which people increase their assets and attributes to gain more power over their lives and has the explicit intent of bringing about social and political change, usually by affecting public policies, decision-making authority and resource allocation.

Community participation	Community development	Community capacity
Can be described as a process by which people become involved in issues in which they share a common concern or need. People can increase their assets and attributes during this process but this is not carried out in a systematic way or even stated as an intended outcome.	Can be described as a process by which outside agencies intentionally build assets and attributes to improve the lives and health of others, linked to economic, social, infrastructural and political opportunities. However, social and political change is not a stated aim or outcome of the process.	Can be described as a process by which outside agencies and people intentionally and systematically build their assets and attributes to improve their lives and health. This is achieved through the use of specific approaches. Like community development, social and political change is not a stated aim or outcome of the process.

be viewed as a process. However, while participation is an interaction between people, for example attending a meeting or a social event, it does not include a commitment towards achieving goals. Action-orientated concepts involve the identification, planning and resolution of community concerns through specified goals and actions. The distinction is also made between participation, action and community empowerment. The key difference between community empowerment and the other community-based concepts is the sense of struggle and liberation that is bound in the process of capacity-building and gaining power. A brief interpretation of each community-based concept is provided in Table 2.2.

The analogy of a 'ladder of community-based interaction' (see Figure 2.1 on p. 23) is used as a framework to clarify the differences between concepts that concern participation, action and empowerment. Sheryl Arnstein (1969) was an early commentator on the use of the rungs of a ladder in her discussion of one concept, citizen participation. Other ideas, for example the 'pyramid diagram' developed for community work in Newcastle, England (Bailey 1991) have been used to show a continuum of activities with increasing degrees of community influence. Here I elaborate upon these ideas to include a discussion of contemporary community-based concepts and illustrate this with examples taken from practice.

Community-based interaction

As communities move toward social and organizational interaction they become more concerned about, and ready to address, the broader determinants on the lives of their members. Understanding the way in which community-based interaction works is an important conceptual tool for the planning, implementation and evaluation of health promotion programmes. Careful consideration needs to be given to the interpretation of community-based concepts in programme planning so that they are correctly used in context, for example the practice of substituting the meaning of community empowerment for the meaning of community participation. This sometimes happens because of their overlapping characteristics but can also be because the concept of participation offers a form of interaction that implies involvement but does not commit the outside agency to help their clients to gain power.

It is important for practitioners to understand the difference between those concepts that involve participation and those that involve action. The key point is that at some stage communities are no longer just passive participants but that people take an active role in identifying and resolving their own concerns. It is also important for practitioners to understand the difference between those concepts that involve action and those that involve

Table 2.2   An interpretation of community-based concepts

Community-based concept	Author's interpretation
Community readiness	A state of community preparedness to engage in a series of stages and a partnership with an outside agent to implement a programme.
Community participation	People become actively involved in a broad range of common needs by sharing their ideas and experiences to identify concerns. Participation is often based on representation as it is not usually possible for all community members to be involved in this process.
Community engagement	People identify problem-solving solutions to issues that affect their lives. This is a collaborative process, often between an outside agency and the community, involving the formation of partnerships that help mobilize resources, influence systems and change relationships.
Community organization	Ability of communities to structure and mobilize themselves toward shared goals. People become involved in shared decision-making and problem-solving that is based on their own self-determination.
Community development	A process by which outside agencies assist communities to improve their lives, often linked to the distribution of resources and to economic, infrastructural and political opportunities as well as to social development.
Community capacity	A systematic approach to build the assets and attributes of communities within a programme context. Uses strategies that 'unpack' this complex concept into its areas of influence or 'domains'.
Community action	A process of ownership by communities of the issues that concern them. The resolution of these issues through participation, capacity-building and community development.
Community empowerment	A process by which communities gain control over the decisions and resources that influence their lives, including the determinants of health. The key difference is the sense of struggle and liberation that is bound in this process of gaining power.

Action

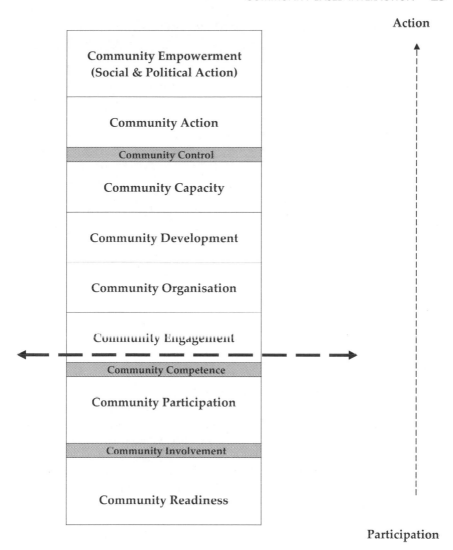

Participation

Figure 2.1 A ladder of community-based interaction

community empowerment. The key point is that at some stage communities will want to address the broader and underlying causes of their powerlessness and will want to become engaged in politically-orientated activities.

This presents three different roles for practitioners in the way in which they work. The first is when the practitioner is directive, instructing communities on what they should do. The second is when the practitioner plays a facilitating role, asking and assisting communities to do what they want towards self-directed goals. The third is when the practitioner works with the community to bring about social and political changes in favour of its members. This role is explicitly a political activity rather than just being goal-orientated.

The 'ladder of community-based interaction' provides one interpretation of what, in practice, is a dynamic and often complicated process. The rungs of the ladder do not represent a linear or chronological progression but they are intended to add clarity to the interaction of a complex set of concepts. The concepts discussed do not actually exist 'out there' in civil society. They have been developed over time in an attempt to explain how communities operate, sometimes based on anecdotal experience and sometimes via more systematic means such as research studies.

The ladder of community-based interaction

The ladder of community-based interaction provides a framework from community readiness, to participation, to engagement, organization, development, capacity-building, collective action and community empowerment. Next is an explanation of each rung on the ladder.

Readiness

Community readiness is a state of community preparedness to engage in a partnership with an outside agent to implement a programme. To reach this state, communities move through a series of stages to develop and implement effective programmes. The measure of preparedness is not the level of ease or difficulty with which the changes from one stage to another are made but the readiness or unreadiness to accept the change (Plested *et al.* 2003). Community readiness implies a willingness to interact but not a previous history of participation between the members of the community. Community readiness does not itself build interaction and is typically measured by an outside agency using questionnaires and interviews to obtain information.

Participation

Community participation builds the interaction of people so that they can address a broad range of common needs by sharing their ideas and experiences (Rifkin 1990). In practice, participation is essentially representation of the majority by a few members of the community. This is because it is not usually possible for everyone to participate in, for example, meetings or workshops. Representation may be through an elected individual who attends a meeting or through a written and signed submission to a committee. As discussed earlier in this chapter, the diversity of individuals and groups within a community can create problems with regard to the selection of representation by its members. Without addressing the redistribution of power, both within and beyond the community, participation can become empty and frustrating for those whose involvement is passive or what Arnstein (1969) called 'non-participation'. It allows those who hold power, those in authority, to claim that all sides were considered while only a few benefit, and this helps to maintain the status quo to their advantage.

UNICEF (1977) was one of the first commentators on community involvement as a form of participation and this concept was developed to explain a way in which to mobilize resources and to facilitate the accessibility of health services. Like participation, this was viewed as a process that could be enhanced through the 'involvement' of the people for which the services were designed (Palmer and Anderson 1986). Participation is also closely linked to community competence and community cohesiveness, concepts that reflect a collective ability for interaction and connectedness between community members (Eng and Parker 1994).

Engagement

Community engagement takes participation a step further by including people in identifying problem-solving solutions to issues that affect their lives. There are many models of community engagement, for example the consultation–public participation model, the asset-based social economy model, the community–democracy model and the community–organizing model (Hashagen 2002). It is a collaborative process, often involving an outside agency (such as an NGO) and the community, and includes the following steps: listening and communication; participation; needs assessment; and working together in partnerships.

Listening and communication
Community engagement begins with people becoming better informed about issues that affect them and how they can become personally involved in addressing them. A lack of understanding regarding, for example, accident and injury prevention can be addressed by having clearer and more accurately targeted information. Listening and communication is more than just informing community members about issues and using one-way channels such as the mass media to provide information.

Participation
Participation, as discussed earlier, is basic to community engagement because it allows people to become involved in activities which influence their lives and health. However, while individuals are able to influence the direction and

implementation of a programme, this alone does not constitute community engagement. Engagement also aims to build community capacities, skills and competencies to enable people to make decisions for themselves and to take appropriate actions. One opportunity for the outside agency to involve the community is through meetings or forums to discuss issues that are important to its members and to disseminate information.

The meeting or forum would typically begin with a brief outline of its purpose followed by an introduction of the participants. The meeting is a facilitated group discussion to focus on a particular issue or community need such as transport, employment and housing. The meeting can be supported by audio-visual materials such as a poster or a video to generate discussion – for example, on the prevention of domestic accidents. The meeting can be used to plan for actions, identify resources, identify potential partners and for people to openly express their views.

Needs assessment
The identification of needs, solutions and actions to resolve the need in regard to, for example, accidents at work, must be carried out by the community. The success of a programme depends to a great extent on the commitment and involvement of the intended beneficiaries. People are much more likely to be committed if they have a sense of ownership in regard to the needs and solutions being addressed by the programme.

Outside agents obviously do often have new and useful information to offer community members. However, this information should not be imposed over the knowledge that resides among community members themselves. The best approach is to use a 'facilitated dialogue' between the community and the outside agents to allow the knowledge and priorities of both to decide an appropriate direction for the programme. Needs assessment undertaken by community members can also strengthen their role in the design of the programme. Programmes that do not address community needs and that do not involve the community in the process of needs assessment usually do not achieve their purpose.

Working together in partnerships
Community links with the outside agency imply an equal partnership based on mutual respect, trust and a sharing of information and experiences. Community links with other people and organizations also include coalitions and alliances. The role of the outside agency is to help community-based organizations to develop partnerships with others who share their needs and concerns. Partnerships build the ability of the community to develop relationships with different groups or organizations based on a recognition of overlapping or mutual interests, and interpersonal and interorganizational respect. They also build the ability to network, collaborate, cooperate and

develop relationships that promote a heightened interdependency among members. Working in partnership will lead toward greater political and social influence of individuals and groups through an expanded membership and resource base – for example, this might involve the development of pressure groups to advocate for changes in legislation.

At this rung of the ladder (marked on Figure 2.1 as a dotted horizontal line) communities are no longer just passive participants. From this point forward, community-based interaction is concerned with people having an active role in identifying the issue to be addressed and the actions by which to resolve these issues. Community-based interaction progresses from being participatory to a more systematic and action-orientated.

Organization

A community that is action-orientated is able to organize and mobilize itself toward shared goals. Through community organization people take a role in shared decision-making and problem-solving that is based on their own self-determination (Braithwaite *et al.* 1994). Historically, the concept of organizing communities was developed, from the programme planner's point of view, to explain a way that people could decrease disease and increase their quality of life. But the root of community organization is based on the work of Saul Alinsky (1972), whose underlying philosophy was that the people should be in control of their own lives. Community organization was a means to empowerment through a number of factors including better leadership, resource mobilization and interpersonal relationships. Organization and development, linked to a collective struggle, became seen by those working with communities as a legitimate model to improve the health and lives of communities.

Development

Community development takes the earlier rungs of the ladder a step further by providing a means by which outside agencies can enable communities to improve their lives. This is through activities and interventions such as education, skills training and technical support. Community development is often linked to the distribution of resources and to economic, infrastructural and political opportunities as well as to social development (Labonte 1998). Community development is designed to include communities in the identification and reinforcement of those aspects of their lives which improve health. It is often an aspect of state policy and therefore remains enmeshed within the dominance of top-down programmes and power-over structures (Petersen 1994). For example, community development includes neighbourhood-based projects that are set up with government support, including an appointed community worker, to address issues of local concern (Jones and Sidell 1997).

Jan Smithies and Georgina Webster (1998: 94) provide a case study of a community development project called the Hutson Street Health Project in Bradford, England. The project covered a deprived inner-city area and was established to work on community health through a number of inter-connecting approaches, such as establishing networks and group activities. An evaluation of the project found that community interaction was built up through small group activities such as cooking and exercise classes, a credit union and a playgroup for children. The project was steered by the expressed needs and involvement of the community but facilitated by a practitioner. The project allowed the community to develop its own action plans and activities for implementation as well as being involved in the day-to-day running of the project, and was funded as part of a broader government initiative toward community development.

Capacity

Community capacity was developed more recently (Goodman *et al.* 1998) than community development to provide a systematic approach to build the assets and attributes of a community within the design of a programme. This has been possible because of the advances made in interpreting this complex concept. The 'domains' of community capacity, similar to community empowerment, are those areas of influence that allow communities to better organize and mobilize themselves toward social and political change. The 'domains' include: participation; leadership; problem assessment; critical reflection; organizational structures; resource mobilization; links to others; programme management; and the role of the outside agent. Community capacity and community empowerment are two overlapping processes (see Table 2.1) that use the 'domains approach' to build more capable communities.

Action

Whereas community capacity builds the assets and attributes of people, community action is the resolution of their concerns to take specific actions to achieve self-identified goals. Communities have ownership of the issues that concern them (Boutilier 1993) and control who identifies the issues to be addressed in a programme. Together, community action and community control are the basis for self-determination that gives people the purpose and direction to improve their lives. Community action often begins when people come together to address local concerns, for example, public transport needs, for short-term periods of time. These groups can also form associations such as NIMBYs ('not in my back yard') directed at local issues that require commitment, for example, the development of a new road that would spoil the natural beauty of their environment. To achieve their actions communities must possess the necessary resources, the attributes discussed on earlier rungs of the ladder and the preparedness to engage with outside agencies. At this point communities have reached a state of self-determination and control and are focused on achieving goals through their own actions.

Empowerment

The key difference between community empowerment and the other community-based concepts is the sense of struggle and liberation that is bound in the process of gaining power. Power cannot be given and must be gained or seized by those who want it against those in authority. Community empowerment is therefore a process by which communities gain more control over the decisions and resources that influence their lives, including the determinants of health. Community empowerment builds from the individual to the group to a wider collective and embodies the intention to bring about social and political change. This is achieved in favour of the 'community' through the redistribution of power, for example, via improved access to resources or decision-making.

There are many examples of community empowerment and here I give a brief outline of a case study in a small town in Australia. Werribee is situated in an agricultural and market gardening area close to the city of Melbourne. In 1996 the local government minister announced the siting of a toxic waste dump at Werribee and Colonial Sugar Refining (CSR) were commissioned by the government to prepare an environmental effects statement with the intention of CSR becoming the implementing agent for the project. The announcement of the siting of the dump was a sufficient emotional trigger for outraged residents to take personal action. Their focus was against the toxic waste dump which residents felt would be detrimental to the health and economy of the community. Individuals quickly organized themselves into a resident's action group called 'WRATD' (Werribee Residents Against Toxic Dump). Local leaders soon emerged who would become instrumental in the development of this 'community of interest' and its rapid growth into a proficient organization. Within a period of 18 months the 'community of interest' had succeeded in establishing an effective campaign to raise public awareness and influence political decision-makers. WRATD employed local experts who gave weight to a sophisticated approach of information dissemination, for example, a computerized operations centre and partnerships with the local university helped to broaden WRATD's expertise. The campaign was carried out in a positive and pervasive manner, constantly working behind the scenes to bring about political and social change in favour of the

Werribee residents. After an enormous show of strength by 15,000 residents, who demonstrated against the siting of the dump, and a petition of more than 100,000 signatures, CSR abandoned the project (Strong 1998 in Laverack 2004: 56).

The overlap between community-based concepts lies in how and why people interact. The similarity lies in the process that people follow from the individual, to groups, to 'communities of interest' and to civil society. The difference often lies in the intended purpose or outcome. The purpose may simply be the participation of people. This interaction may later become more concerned with building the competencies and capacities of people. Alternatively, the interaction may become more directed toward specific goals and actions. But only when these goals are directed at social and political change do communities begin to empower themselves. If properly applied, community-based concepts can help health promotion practitioners to better understand the way in which communities operate. They can also help practitioners to appreciate the role that they have in facilitating community participation, action and empowerment in their everyday work.

Chapter 3 discusses the link between health and empowerment and explains how, as practitioners, we can address the determinants of health through health promotion practice.

3 Health and empowerment

This chapter begins with an interpretation of the different meanings of health and then provides a discussion of the link between empowerment and improved health outcomes. The chapter also examines the link between the determinants of health and health inequality, and the relevance of this to health promotion practice.

Interpreting the meaning of health

The meaning of 'health' can be interpreted in multiple ways. The way in which individuals, for example, interpret the meaning of their own health is a personal experience. Health is subjective and its interpretation is relative to the environment and culture in which people live. Health can mean different things to different people. People can define health in functional terms by their ability to carry out certain roles and responsibilities rather than the absence of disease. People are concerned with the trade-offs they have to make in order to gain their own interpretation of good health. For example, people who are diseased or ill may still perceive themselves as being healthy and willing to bear discomfort and pain because it does not outweigh the inconvenience, loss of control or financial cost of having the condition treated (Cohen and Henderson 1991). Individual interpretations of health are complex and interrelated to a person's self-esteem, level of social support, individual control and social status. A review of heart health inequalities in Canada, for example, found that people who experience low income, less control in their lives and a poor education are more likely to experience morbidity and mortality. The higher one's position in the workplace or society, the greater one's power (control), wealth and status, the better one's health and sense of self-esteem (Labonte 1993).

The World Health Organization (WHO) definition of health has become one of the most commonly used official interpretations in health promotion. This definition was first included in the preamble to the *Constitution of the World Health Organization* as adopted by the International Health Conference, New York, 19–22 June 1946, signed on 22 July 1946 by the representatives of 61 states and entered into force on 7 April 1948. The WHO definition has not been amended since 1948: 'Health is a state of complete physical, mental and social well-being and not merely the absence of disease or infirmity' (WHO 2006).

Physical well-being is concerned with the healthy functioning of the body, biological normality, physical fitness and capacity to perform tasks. Social well-being includes interpersonal relationships as well as wider social issues such as marital satisfaction, employability and community involvement. Mental well-being involves self-efficacy, subjective well-being and social inclusion and is the ability of a person to adapt to their environment and the society in which they function (Laverack 2004). The WHO definition, as an ideal state of physical, social and mental well-being, is a positive interpretation of health and has been criticized for not taking other dimensions into account, namely the emotional and spiritual aspects of health (Ewles and Simnett 2003).

Official and personal interpretations of health can be significantly different from one another. It is important to remember that both are ideal types and in practice they coexist together and inform one another. Practitioners have embraced official interpretations because they are measurable and accountable. This being the case, the measurement of health has focused on the biomedical approach that is concerned with demonstrating a relationship between a health status measure (such as cancer) and a specific behaviour (such as smoking). Consequently, a health promotion practice that uses interpretations of illness and disease, rather than the way in which people view their own health, largely implements programmes aimed at reducing morbidity and mortality. These programmes are delivered in a top-down, power-over style that maintains control with an outside agency that is concerned with accountability and quantifiable effectiveness.

The link between empowerment and improved health outcomes

In the community psychology literature, empowerment is seen to enhance individual competence and self-esteem. This in turn increases perceptions of personal control and has a direct effect on improving health outcomes (Wallerstein 1992). This argument can be extended to include an individual's connectedness with other people and their participation in groups and communities of interest who wish to gain more power, with the intent of bringing about changes in their external environment (Zimmerman and Rappaport 1988).

In the community health literature, empowerment is generally viewed as a process beginning with individual action and then progressing to the development of small mutual groups, community organizations, partnerships and ultimately social and political action (Labonte 1990). The zero-sum form of power is most commonly seen to exist in a culture of health promotion programming that is based on finite resources. The community health literature recognizes that many of the inequalities in health are a result of power relations that have an effect on the distribution of resources and the development of policy. Social and structural changes can be brought about by people attaining the power they need to redress inequalities and community empowerment is often the process they use to achieve this (Laverack 2005).

Community-based empowerment initiatives that lead to improvements in health outcomes have focused largely on environmental changes. These often have an immediate impact on behaviours that are measurable during the time period covered by the intervention (Carr 2000). The evidence shows that community action has been able to lead to sustained changes in the social and organizational environment, linked to improvements in health in, for example, alcohol abuse and injury prevention. Community action in Surfers Paradise, Australia, led to increased regulation of licensed alcohol premises and the implementation of policies and a code of practice for bar staff, and as a consequence reduced alcohol-related violence (Homel *et al.* 1997; Hauritz *et al.* 1998). Community action at Piha, New Zealand, resulted in bans on public drinking, leading to fewer injuries and incidents of crime and an improved sense of well-being (Conway 2002). Elsewhere, community action projects on alcohol regulation have resulted in bar staff training, shortening of hours of operation of licensed premises, increased age verification checks and highly visible drink driving enforcement, resulting in reductions in injury (Holder *et al.* 1997) and in drink driving in those aged 18–19 years (Wagenaar *et al.* 2000).

Nina Wallerstein, a prominent academic and advocate for community empowerment, has also found distinct links between empowerment and health outcomes. Her review of the literature (Wallerstein 2006) found that empowerment strategies are promising in their ability to produce both empowerment and health impacts. The literature shows a consistency of empowerment strategies and outcomes at the psychological, organizational, and community levels, and across multiple populations, though specific outcomes vary by issue and societal context. Empowerment strategies are more likely to be successful if integrated within macroeconomic and political policy strategies aimed at creating greater equity. In the light of the evidence available and other information accessible, empowerment strategies are promising in working with socially excluded populations. While participatory processes are at the base of empowerment, participation alone is insufficient if strategies do not also build the capacity to challenge non-responsive or oppressive institutions and to redress power imbalances.

Effective empowerment strategies depend as much on the agency and leadership of the people involved as the overall context in which they take place. Health promotion programmes that plan to use empowerment strategies to improve health outcomes should consider the following.

1   Integrate empowerment strategies that have been shown to be most effective into the overall design of the programme, for example:

- increasing citizens' skills, access to information and resources;
- use of small group efforts which enhance critical consciousness to build supportive environments and a deeper sense of community;
- promoting community action through collective involvement in decision-making and participation in all phases of planning, implementation, and evaluation; use of lay helpers/leaders; advocacy and leadership training; and organizational and coalition capacity development;
- strengthening healthy public policy through organizational and interorganizational actions; transfer of power and decision-making authority to participants of interventions; and promoting/demanding transparency and accountability of government and other institutions;
- having community members define and act on community needs, including as health consumers.

2   Build on other successful strategies especially for marginalized populations such as youth, those at risk for HIV/AIDS, women, and the poor. These strategies support participation which promotes autonomy and decision-making authority; a sense of community and social interaction and power from within, which can lead to a change in people's circumstances.

3   Build on successful patient and family caregiver strategies to reorient health services so patients and families are seen as resources with the capacity to be partners in improving their health.

4   Foster the refinement of measurement tools on empowerment domains.

5   Foster training for health and development aid professionals, service providers, policy-makers and community leaders on community empowerment strategies, community-based participatory research and participatory evaluation (Wallerstein 2006).

There is more evidence to show the pathways through which the link between empowerment and health outcomes occur within a programming context. These pathways have been identified as the areas of influence or 'domains' of community empowerment (Laverack 2001). The domains represent those aspects of the process of community empowerment that allow individuals and groups to organize and mobilize themselves toward social and political change. The empowerment domains are: participation; organizational structures; local leadership; resource mobilization; asking 'why';

problem assessment; links with other people and organizations; and the role of outside agents and programme management. The domains are robust and provide a useful means to unpack the concept of community empowerment and to demonstrate the link it has to health outcomes. The evidence for the link between each empowerment 'domain' and specific improved health outcomes includes the following (Laverack 2006b).

Participation and improved health outcomes

There are few studies that have been able to measure the health benefits of community participation. However, individuals do have a better chance of achieving their health goals if they can participate with other people who are affected by the same or similar circumstances to build interpersonal trust and trust in public institutions (Brehm and Rahn 1997). For example, the use of participatory learning exercises in women's groups in a poor rural population in Nepal led to a reduction in neonatal and maternal mortality (Manandhar *et al.* 2004). The women in the intervention clusters were found to have antenatal care, institutional delivery, trained birth attendance and more hygienic care and this led to an improvement in birth outcomes. By participating in groups the women were better able to define, analyse and then, through the support of others, articulate and act on their concerns around childbirth. The advantage of participation was that it strengthened social networks and improved social support between the women and between the women and the providers of health service delivery.

Participation in groups that share interests can help individuals to compete for limited resources and increase the sense of personal control in their lives. For example, the link between psychological empowerment (power from within) in patients and health has been demonstrated in several recent studies (Everson *et al.* 1997; Odedina *et al.* 2000; Lupton *et al.* 2005).

Organizational structures and improved health outcomes

Community organizations provide the opportunity for their members to gain the skills and competencies that are necessary to allow them to move toward achieving health outcomes. On an individual basis this includes self-help groups that provide knowledge, skills and social support around issues such as smoking cessation, dieting and exercise classes. On a collective and organizational basis these skills include planning and strategy development, team-building, networking, negotiation, fundraising, marketing and proposal writing. In Box 3.1 I provide an example of empowerment for health outcomes in women's groups in Western Samoa.

Box 3.1 Empowerment for health outcomes in Samoa

A national programme designed to address women's health needs in Western Samoa, Polynesia, created a community-based self-help network based on neighbourhood support and nursing care that operated through existing women's health committees (WHCs). The WHCs were prestigious organizations and were well attended by all women. The government supported the development of these community organizations through resource allocation, training and regular visits from health workers. The purpose was to develop the skills and competencies of their members in the areas of child care, weaning practices and sanitation, which had been previously identified as the main causes of infant mortality. Each WHC put into force village health regulations relating to sanitation to which all families had to conform. The programme not only brought about improvements in women's health but also their authority, as well as an improved ability to organize and mobilize themselves and to raise funds for other projects. The WHCs became the largest and most influential group in the community and were increasingly involved in a range of community concerns. The WHCs were based on an ideology of equality and empowerment, but somewhat ironically their success was through the legitimate use of top-down traditional authority (Thomas 2001).

Local leadership and improved health outcomes

An example of the role that local leaders can play in influencing health is given by Lucy Earle, a community development researcher, and her colleagues, regarding a programme in Central Asia (Earle *et al.* 2004: 27). The village leader in one community had used his influence to obtain assistance from an outside organization to help provide irrigation pipes and an electric pump to improve the water supply of the community. But not all members of the community were satisfied with these developments, especially groups of low-income women. The water supplied was too expensive for them and the pipes were laid to better serve the family members of the village leader. However, they could not complain because to contradict the leader could mean serious consequences for the livelihoods of poor families. For example, the village leader provided temporary employment during harvest and distributed flour to poorer residents. Not only did the leader hold an influential position in the community but his sons also held posts in the local government administration. The village leader was able to use his power over others in the community, mostly marginalized groups, to manipulate the distribution of resources and gain access to decision-making processes.

Resource mobilization and improved health outcomes

The ability of a community to mobilize resources from within and to ne-gotiate resources from beyond itself is an indication of a developed organi-zational ability, but there is little evidence to suggest that this alone will allow a community to gain social and political power. However, there is evidence to suggest that resource mobilization and improved literacy and education, particularly for women, can lead to improved health outcomes in developing countries (Bratt *et al.* 2002; Pokhrel and Sauerborn 2004).

An example of the link between resource mobilization and improved health is the use of swimming pools in remote Aboriginal communities in Australia. These were found to reduce ear, nose and throat infections (Carapetis *et al.* 1995) and to provide an overall improvement in the well-being of the community (Peart and Szoeke 1998). The public swimming pools in-variably operated at a loss and costs were borne or subsidized by the govern-ment because it was seen as a recreational facility which promoted the health of the population. The people living in the communities had low incomes and access to only limited resources. They were expected by the government to raise finances to maintain the pools. The communities started to raise addi-tional internal resources on a small scale through fundraising and pool ent-rance fees and to raise external resources through other funding sources. In this way, the ability of the community to mobilize resources had an effect on its health through the continued use of the swimming pools (Laverack 2005).

'Asking why' and improved health outcomes

An example of how asking why or critical reflection can influence health outcomes is provided through the use of 'Photovoice' developed by Caroline Wang and her colleagues (Wang *et al.* 1998). Photovoice is a process by which people can identify, represent and enhance their community through a spe-cific photographic technique. It entrusts cameras to the hands of people to enable them to act as recorders, and potential catalysts for social action and change, in their own communities. It uses the immediacy of the visual image and accompanying stories to furnish evidence and to promote an effective, participatory means of sharing expertise to create healthy public policy.

Communities using Photovoice engage in a three-stage process that provides the foundation for analysing the pictures they have taken.

- *Stage 1, selecting* – choosing those photographs that most accurately reflect the community's concerns and assets. So that people can lead the discussion, it is they who choose the photographs. They select photographs they consider most significant, or simply like best, from each roll of film they have taken.

- *Stage 2, contextualizing* – telling stories about what the photographs mean. The participatory approach also generates the second stage, contextualizing or storytelling. This occurs in the process of group discussion, suggested by the acronym VOICE: voicing our individual and collective experience. Photographs alone, considered outside the context of their own voices and stories, contradict the essence of Photovoice. People describe the meaning of their images in small and large group discussions.

- *Stage 3, codifying* – identifying the issues, themes or theories that emerge. The participatory approach gives multiple meanings to singular images and thus frames the third stage, codifying. In this stage, participants may identify three types of dimension that arise from the dialogue process: issues, themes, or theories. The individual or group may codify issues when the concerns targeted for action are pragmatic, immediate and tangible. This is the most direct application of the analysis. The individual or group may also codify themes and patterns, or develop theories that are grounded in a more systematic analysis of the images (Photovoice 2006).

Box 3.2 provides an example of how Photovoice has been used to strengthen maternal and child health.

Box 3.2 Photovoice for maternal and child health

This Photovoice project took place in Contra Costa, a large economically and ethnically diverse county in the San Francisco Bay area. Sixty county residents aged 13–50 participated in three sessions during which they received training from the local health department in the techniques and process of Photovoice. Residents were provided with disposable cameras and were encouraged to take photographs reflecting their views on family, maternal and child health (MCH) assets and concerns in their community, and then participated in group discussions about their photographs. Community events were held to enable participants to educate MCH staff and community leaders.

The photovoice project provided MCH staff with information to supplement existing quantitative perinatal data and contributed to an understanding of key MCH issues that participating community residents wanted to see addressed. Participants' concerns centred on the need for safe places for children's recreation and for improvement in the broader community environment within county neighbourhoods. Participants' definitions of family and MCH assets and concerns differed from those of MCH professionals (typically, low birth weight, maternal mortality and teen pregnancy prevention), and this helped MCH staff to expand their priorities and include residents' foremost concerns.

MCH professionals applied Photovoice as an innovative participatory research methodology to engage community members in needs assessment, asset mapping and programme planning, and to reach policy-makers to advocate strategies promoting family and MCH as informed from a grassroots perspective (Wang and Pies 2004).

Problem assessment and improved health outcomes

Addressing health outcomes does not necessarily start with the community tackling health problems but may cover a range of personal, social, economic and environmental factors. The key issue is that practitioners must be prepared to listen to what the members of the community want. They may not necessarily like what they hear, but they must be committed to moving forward and building upon these issues. The motivation to improve health must come from within the community and cannot come from an outside 'expert'. Programme inputs such as education and training can play a role in improving health outcomes but these must always support the problems that have been identified by the community as being relevant to their needs (Syme 1997).

An example is a health programme in India working to improve the lives of rural women in Gujarat. The women first requested and then received cooking stoves that would reduce the level of smoke in their small, airless huts. Finding a solution to this initial problem led the women to go on and identify other health-related problems in their community including poor maternal and child health facilities and the gynaecological training of health workers (Rifkin 2003).

Links with others and improved health outcomes

Links with others demonstrates the ability to develop relationships outside the community, often based on mutual interests. The development of partnerships is an important step toward empowerment and can also lead to an improvement in health outcomes by pooling limited resources and by taking collective action.

The Asian Health Forum in Liverpool, England, identified a large number of cases of depression and isolation among Asian women in the area. A health worker held discussions with them and then approached a leisure centre to arrange swimming lessons. This arrangement would ensure privacy – for example, windows would be blacked out and the lessons run by other women. The alliance, between the Asian women and the leisure centre, was able to organize weekly lessons and to secure funding for a female instructor. The lessons were very popular and timings had to be reorganized to avoid conflict with other pool activities and to accommodate the young children of the

Asian swimmers. The lessons had a health benefit to the women by helping to reduce weight but mostly through an improved feeling of well-being brought about by regular exercise. Eventually the health worker was able to delegate some of the responsibility for the lessons to the alliance and slowly their interest moved to other sports activities and resulted in an increase in the choices available to Asian women (Jones and Sidell 1997).

The role of the outside agents and improved health outcomes

Health promotion practice is traditionally professionally led, for example, it is the practitioner or their agency that chooses the individuals, groups and communities that they will work with and the methods to be used. The initiation of the empowerment process and the enthusiasm for its direction and progress is also often professionally led. Practitioners, who are in a position of relative power, work to help others who are in a relatively powerless position to gain more control.

Individual control, in part a consequence of the position of people in structural and social hierarchies, has been shown to have an influence on their health and well-being. In a programme context the issue becomes how much control the outside agent (the practitioner or agency) gives to the community for thre programme's design, implementation, management, evaluation, finances and administration. The community must have a sense of ownership of the programme, which in turn must address their concerns.

An example of this is provided by the health authority in Oldham, United Kingdom, which established a 'local voices' steering group with the purpose of involving local people in health activities. The group was made up of representatives from different departments, community trusts and government agencies in a poor housing area. The group decided to employ an independent consultant to carry out a participatory needs assessment. The community members were invited to attend meetings to express their concerns. Child care facilities and transport were arranged and meetings were held at times that would be convenient to the community. Large meetings were often followed by small group discussions to elicit further information from the community about what they felt affected their health. These initial discussions led to the development of a questionnaire which was administered on a door-to-door basis by trained interviewers. This process involved a relationship between different representatives working and living in the community to coordinate the activities of an outside agent, the consultants, to provide a specific technical input (Smithies and Webster 1998). The important issue is that the outside agents were able to collect information in a way that was acceptable to all representatives and this allowed the community to take the necessary action to effect change.

Empowering people to address the determinants of health

A notable difference in the definition of health promotion in two key documents, the *Ottawa Charter* (WHO 1986) and the *Bangkok Charter* (WHO 2005) is the link with the determinants of health. The *Bangkok Charter* acknowledges the importance of the determinants of health and states that 'health promotion is the process of enabling people to increase control over their health and its determinants' (WHO 2005: 1). The determinants of health gained prominence in the period after the development of the *Ottawa Charter* and are the range of personal, economic and environmental factors which determine the health status of individuals or populations. A fuller discussion on the determinants of health can be found in Marmot and Wilkinson (1999), covering their lifelong importance in regard to the following (Wilkinson 2003).

- *The social gradient*: life expectancy is shorter for people further down the social ladder, who are likely to experience twice as much disease and ill health as those nearer the top in society. This influence also affects people across society – for example, within middle-class office workers those with lower-ranking jobs experience more disease.
- *Stress*: people who are worried, anxious and unable to psychologically cope suffer from stress that over long periods of time can damage their health – for example, high blood pressure, stroke or depression – and may lead to premature death. Stress can result from many different circumstances in a person's life but the lower people are in the social gradient the more common are these problems.
- *Early life*: slow physical growth and poor emotional support can result in a lifetime of poor health and a reduced psychological functioning in adulthood. Poor foetal development, linked to, for example, stress, addiction and poor prenatal care is a risk for health in later life.
- *Social exclusion*: poverty, discrimination and racism can all contribute to social exclusion. These processes all prevent people from participating in health and education services, are psychologically damaging and can lead to illness and premature death.
- *Work*: while having a job is generally healthier than not having a job, stress in the workplace increases the risk of ill health – for example, back pain, sickness absence and cardiovascular disease. This is more pronounced when people have little opportunity to use their skills and have low decision-making authority.
- *Unemployment*: job security increases health, unemployment or the insecurity of losing one's job can cause illness and premature death.

The health effects of unemployment are linked to psychological factors such as anxiety brought on by problems of debt.

* *Social support*: having friends, good social relationships and supportive networks can improve health. People have better health when they feel cared for, loved, esteemed and valued. Conversely, people who do not have these factors in their lives suffer from poorer health and premature death.
* *Addiction*: alcohol dependence, illicit drug use and smoking are not only markers of social and economic disadvantage but are also important factors in worsening health. People can enter into addictive relationships to provide a temporary release from the pain of harsh social and economic conditions and stress, but as a result their long-term health is damaged.
* *Food*: a good diet and an adequate supply of food are important to health and well-being. A poor diet can cause malnutrition and a variety of deficiencies that can contribute to, for example, cancer and diabetes and can also lead to obesity. Poor diet is often associated with people who are lower on the social gradient.
* *Transport*: reliance on mechanized transport has resulted in people taking less exercise, increased fatal accidents and pollution. Other forms of transport such as cycling and walking increase the level of exercise and help people to reduce obesity and diseases such as diabetes and heart disease.

People who have high-risk lifestyles or who have poor living conditions are typically influenced by economic and political policies and practices and have more disease, a higher risk of premature death and less well-being (Wilkinson 2003). The determinants of health provide a helpful guide to the specific areas were people's lives can be influenced by policies and practices.

Next is a description of my early life experiences to illustrate the factors that influence the everydayness of the determinants of health.

This boy's life: the everydayness of the determinants of health

I was born the first child to working-class parents. My father was a lorry driver and my mother was a cleaner. Both my parents smoked and drank alcohol and I was born premature and low birth weight, spending the first two weeks of my life in a hospital incubator. When I left hospital we lived in rented accommodation, my mother breastfed me and I quickly grew into an active toddler. We had a typical English working-class diet of fatty foods, low in fibre, high in sugar, and a lack of variety in what we ate. We relied on government support for our health and dental care and as a 5–7-year-old child I suffered from a variety of chronic illnesses including dental caries, ear, nose and eye infections, fevers and throat infections. My mother sometimes could not find time to take me to a dentist or doctor and so ailments were simply ignored until they became more serious. The result was that I had to periodically take time off school to recover my health.

My parents argued a lot and this created a stressful home environment. As an only child I did not have anyone else in the family to provide social support and therefore spent more and more time away from home with the families of other children. At the age of 7 my circumstances worsened. My parents separated. My mother and I moved to live somewhere else far away from my father, first to another family (this was crowded and stressful and I felt unwanted) and then to a very small house. The house had no heating, no internal toilet or bathroom and was damp.

At my new school I found it difficult to make new friends. It was full of working-class kids, many just like myself, being raised in difficult circumstances at the lower end of society. The school staff did not have the capacity to cope with or even identify my learning disability. I suffered from a form of dyslexia and this was not diagnosed because I did not have access to proper educational facilities. As a result my school record was poor and I was placed in a class with other 'problem' or 'slow' students. Many of my classmates played truant because they too were fed up with their lessons or with being treated as stupid by their teachers. Out of school my friends got into mischief which often involved damaging property or petty theft. By the age of 10, I was in trouble with the police and became labelled as a 'troublemaker' and a 'poor student' with family problems. I became an obvious target for the frustrations of the system and families higher up the social gradient as someone responsible for antisocial behaviour. I was socially excluded from events in which other children took part. People thought that I had no future and would end up unemployed or in prison.

My mother had to work in two low-paid jobs to support us but the household income was still lower than when we were with my father. We depended on other people and even more than before on what government support we could get. There was no extra money to run a car, to buy new clothes or to go on holiday. By 12 I was the typical 'latchkey kid', playing on the streets until late at night and coming home to let myself into the house and to go to bed while my mother had to work in a bar. Still, we survived as a family and most of my childhood memories are good and happy ones. We had a network of, and the support of, friends, some of whom were in a similar position to my mother, raising children by themselves. Our kitchen became a meeting place where people could come for a cup of tea and a chat about their problems of domestic violence, drinking and debt. Stress, addictions, social exclusion, unemployment and a low social status were a part of everyday life.

Did my circumstances lead to inequality? Did my circumstances damage my health? Both as an individual and as part of a family unit I had little choice or control over my circumstances. My mother and myself lived our lives from day to day, almost from hand to mouth; we did not plan ahead for fear of the unknown and did what other people around us did. Our friends and family were all from the lower part of the social gradient and so were disadvantaged, like we were, by political and economic policies.

My mother and myself did suffer from inequalities in income, in education and in health compared to other families who were higher on the social gradient. These inequalities in health generally took three forms:

1   *Inequalities in access to health care.* Some people have difficulty accessing primary health care services; for example, my mother had to work in two jobs and found it difficult to take me to the clinic for a dental or doctor's appointment.
2   *Inequalities in health outcomes.* Differences in average life expectancy at birth between different socioeconomic groups. For example, my life expectancy was less than for a boy born into a middle-class family with educated parents.
3   *Inequalities in the determinants of health.* Different people have very different experiences of the determinants of health. These different experiences, (such as disability, single parenthood, quality of school, income, age of housing stock, type of road user), can have an effect on health. I went to a poor-quality school, lived in basic housing, relied on public transport and had a single parent. In this situation inequalities become entrenched. When these experiences overlapped they had a 'snowballing' effect and a greater combined impact on my life and the life of my mother.

Medical care has been important in prolonging life and in improving prognosis after a serious illness, but the common causes of ill health that affect populations are social, political, economic and environmental. These determinants reflect the way we live and come and go far quicker than medical-based factors. This is the main reason that life expectancy has improved over recent generations and why some countries have improved the health of their population while others have not. It is also why inequalities in health have increased – for example, the gap between the health of rich and poor social groups has widened (Wilkinson 2003).

The determinants of health are multiple and interactive and health promotion traditionally addresses those factors which are modifiable – for example, behaviours, lifestyles, income and the physical environment (WHO 1998). However, the key to addressing the determinants of, and inequalities in, health is the redistribution of power and by transforming unequal power relationships which are indicative of our society and working practices.

Chapter 4 discusses the nature of health promotion programming and offers an approach that allows empowerment approaches to be accommodated within traditional top-down health promotion programmes.

4 Empowerment and health promotion programming

Health promotion is largely controlled by state departments or government-funded agencies such as NGOs. Health promotion practitioners are employed to deliver information, resources and services and are often seen as an outside agent to the people who are their clients. The practitioner can be an individual, such as a community health nurse, or an organization such as a health department or trust. Their clients cover the range of people who act as the recipients of the information, resources and services being delivered to promote health – for example, individuals, concerned groups of individuals such as residents, and community-based organizations that have been formed to address a specific issue (Laverack 2005).

Health promotion programming is professionally-led and it is the practitioner or their agency that usually chooses the design, the means of implementation and the evaluation of the programme. This includes the selection of 'targeted groups' (the clients) and the methods to be used to reach them. Similarly, the initiation of the programme, the empowerment approaches that it uses and the enthusiasm for its direction are often led by the practitioner. This raises a fundamental constraint in health promotion practice: the issues to be addressed are traditionally identified by an outside agent rather than by individuals, groups or communities.

Health promotion programming entails a power relationship between different stakeholders (see Box 4.1). This is primarily between the practitioner and their agencies, representing the state, and their clients, the people, groups and communities with whom they work 'out there' in civil society. This raises the issue of how practitioners bridge the gap between state and civil society. The practitioners in a programme are in a position of relative power to their clients, who are in a relatively powerless position. It is usually the practitioner who controls the allocation of limited resources, selecting who is to receive skills training, education and advisory services, and they are in a better position to use their 'expert power' to legitimize the concerns of their clients. In this book I argue that a key way to bridge the gap between the state and civil society is for practitioners to engage their clients in approaches with the means of reaching empowered solutions.

> **Box 4.1** Definition of stakeholders
>
> Stakeholders are people, groups and organizations who have some interest or in-fluence in the programme. The primary stakeholders or beneficiaries are those people who are ultimately affected and at whom the programme is usually tar-geted, for example the community. The secondary stakeholders are the people or organizations that act as an intermediary in the delivery of a programme. They are the outside agents – for example health promoters, government or NGOs. An outside agent can also be a primary stakeholder – for example, community health workers who live in the community and who are appointed to manage programme activities at the community level (Laverack 1999).

Health promotion programming and parallel tracking

In practice, health promotion is most commonly implemented as activities set within the context of a programme. This is conventionally managed and monitored by a practitioner and includes: a period of identification; design; appraisal; approval; implementation; management; and evaluation. Ideally, the programme addresses the concerns of the beneficiaries based on discus-sions with the community prior to implementation. The concerns are prior-itized and then developed into a form that makes sense to all the programme stakeholders. The design of the programme reflects the concerns as a clear statement of objectives, identifying in advance suitable indicators of progress and the prior assessment of risks and assumptions.

The way in which health concerns are to be addressed and are defined in a programme is one of the most important issues and can take two distinct forms: 'top-down' and 'bottom-up'. 'Top-down' describes programmes where problem identification comes from those in top structures 'down' to the community. 'Bottom-up' is the reverse, where the community identifies its own problems and communicates these to those who have the decision-making authority. I intentionally use these two terms in this book because they help to illustrate the power relationship that exists in health promotion programming. What should be remembered is that the terms 'top-down' and 'bottom-up' are ideal types of health promotion practice that are used to demonstrate important differences in relation to programme design.

These two types of programming often have different agendas that create a bottom-up versus top-down 'tension'. The practitioner uses their power-over to 'push down' a predefined agenda onto the community through 'vertical' or so called 'siloed' programming. The community attempts to 'push up' an agenda based on their immediate concerns that may not be the same as those identified by the practitioner. Top-down programmes would include almost all health education and multi-risk factor reduction interventions and are the predominant style of health promotion programming. Bottom-up programmes are fewer in design and often exist as a part of larger scale top-down programming. In top-down programming, community empowerment is seen as a lower level objective which is typically centred on improving health or preventing disease through increasing knowledge or by changing behaviours.

The key questions that distinguish between top-down and bottom-up programme design are now discussed.

Does the programme have a fixed timeframe or a flexible timeframe?

Top-down programmes have a fixed and specific timeframe, typically one to three years, to allow the funding agency to plan its technical inputs within expenditure cycles. In contrast, a longer timeframe is necessary to achieve community empowerment, typically five to seven years. Requests for an extension of the timeframe by the community can be viewed by funding agencies as a failure of the programme to meet its objectives. To overcome this issue, the programme should have a more flexible timeframe. Some of the empowerment outcomes may be achieved within a relatively short timeframe of a few months. However, as this cannot always be guaranteed, an evaluation of the process will provide evidence of the success of the 'empowerment track' even within a limited timeframe.

Is it the outside agent or the community who identifies the concerns to be addressed?

Both the outside agent and the community have concerns that they wish to address. The concerns of the outside agent are typically based on top-down procedures that employ positivist forms of data collection such as from epidemiological studies and systematic reviews, for example, reducing the level of obesity in schoolchildren based on an analysis of clinical information from nursing staff. The concerns of communities are typically based on:

- meeting their immediate needs; for example, providing child care facilities; and/or
- addressing issues that have an historical context; for example, concerns raised by residents of the increase of antisocial behaviour by children in their community.

Sometimes the concerns of the outside agent and the community are similar and can be reconciled in the design of the programme. More often, the concerns of the outside agent and the community are dissimilar and a compromise has to be found. This usually involves the needs of the community not being accommodated within the design of a top-down programme.

Parallel tracking allows both sets of concerns to be accommodated into the programme design.

Is it the outside agent or the community who has control over the management of the programme?

Top-down programmes are conventionally managed by an outside agent. The members of the community are expected to cooperate and contribute to the programme under the instruction of the programme management team. Bottom-up approaches consciously involve the community in the management of the programme through skills training and by increasingly devolving responsibility for activities such as planning, report writing, budgeting and evaluation.

How is the programme evaluated?

If evaluation is concerned with targets and outcomes and is carried out by the outside agent or by independent 'experts' it is typically top-down. If evaluation is concerned with capacity-building and processes that actively involve the community it is typically bottom-up. Empowering evaluation uses procedures that are participatory and that involve the community, in order to obtain their input in the process as well as developing their skills in conducting an assessment.

The challenge to practitioners is how they can accommodate community empowerment (bottom-up) approaches within the dominant top-down styles of health promotion programming. This requires a fundamental change in the way we think about health promotion programming. Rather than viewing the issue as a bottom-up versus top-down tension, the process of accommodating community empowerment into top-down programming can be better viewed as a 'parallel track' running along side the main 'programme track' (see Figure 4.1). The tensions between the two styles of programming then occur at each stage of the programme cycle, making their resolution much easier to achieve. Theoretically, this helps to move our thinking on from a simple bottom-up/top-down dichotomy. Practically, it provides a systematic way in which to accommodate the two styles of programming (Laverack 2004).

The main purpose of the programme remains unchanged, with a focus on more conventional top-down issues – for example, disease prevention. This means that the design of the programme fits within the expectations of, and is therefore more acceptable to, governments and funding agencies but still has a clearly defined role for capacity-building and empowerment.

While most health promotion programmes are top-down, those who actively wish to work in more empowering ways remain passionate about the

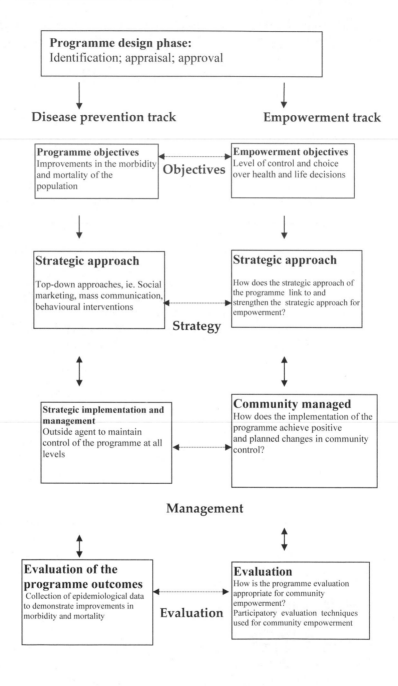

Figure 4.1 Parallel tracking empowerment in chronic disease programmes

potential of health promotion and use bottom-up activities in their everyday work. These empowering activities are often not recognized as an important element of the programme design and may receive insufficient funding. Where empowering approaches are already used as part of the programme design they can be emphasized and built upon by using parallel tracking. Where empowering approaches do not exist as part of the programme design, the structure of parallel tracking alerts the practitioner as to when to include these elements as part of a programme cycle.

Next, I provide a case study of how parallel tracking can be used to accommodate empowerment approaches at each phase of a programme (design, objective-setting, strategic approach, implementation and evaluation) that aims to target Polynesian people at high risk of chronic disease.

Accommodating empowerment approaches into chronic disease programmes

Chronic disease prevention programmes are typically designed to address changes in lifestyle and behaviour centred on, for example, cardiovascular disease, diabetes, obesity and smoking cessation. The health promotion intervention is based on epidemiological evidence and is typically top-down and managed by an outside agent.

Metabolic syndrome (also referred to as 'insulin resistance syndrome' and 'syndrome X') consists of several disorders of the body's metabolism at the same time, including obesity, high blood pressure, diabetes and high cholesterol. This syndrome affects at least one out of every five overweight people and can lead to increased morbidity and mortality from cardiovascular and kidney disease. Health promotion programmes are designed to help people at high risk from metabolic syndrome to change their lifestyle and behaviour in regard to diet and exercise.

In Auckland, New Zealand, Polynesian people aged 45 years and above have rates for cardiovascular and ischaemic heart disease which are consistently and significantly higher (about twice as high) than those in the total population. Polynesian males and females also have higher prevalence rates for diabetes and worse causal-related indicators for obesity, diet, physical exercise and tobacco consumption (Ministry of Health and Ministry of Pacific Island Affairs 2004).

The programme design phase

The key issue is: who will have the power-over (access to resources and decision-making authority) the implementation and management of the programme?

It is at the design phase that the power relationship is established between the practitioner, or their agency, and the other stakeholders of the programme, in particular the intended beneficiaries. Top-down programming is a manifestation of power-over, in which the practitioner exercises control of financial and other material resources of the programme. It is a form of dominance and authority in which control has traditionally been exerted and facilitated through the design of the programme.

Parallel tracking moves the practitioner away from top-down programming to a position in which power-over is shared by all stakeholders. It provides a more precise role for the practitioner, one that helps their clients to gain power and address the concerns that influence their lives and health. At the design phase the practitioner assists their clients to facilitate their involvement to resolve their issues through the programme using their own actions, and identify and rank the issues that are important to them and that will be addressed through the programme. Box 4.2 provides an example of how practitioners can help people to identify and rank their concerns. This process involves more than conducting a community survey, appraisal or consultation to obtain the opinions of a particular 'community of interest'. The purpose is to actively engage with the community, or its representatives, and to give them a voice to express their concerns and needs. This can be identified on a general basis – for example, what are your health concerns? or be specific to the programme – for example, what are your concerns regarding heart disease? With regard to chronic disease in Polynesian peoples these concerns have been identified by Tongan community groups as (Moana 2005):

- Better facilities for vegetable gardening. A good form of exercise and an activity that people wanted to do, especially the aged.
- Walking groups for men and women. A means of also building social networks and support groups based around a physical activity.
- More information about diabetes, in both English and Polynesian languages, presented via different channels of communication.

Box 4.2   Mapping and ranking community concerns

Mapping is a participatory technique to allow individuals and groups to identify and better understand their concerns. It can be carried out using a visual means, for example, a drawing such as a picture, a chart or another form of visual representation such as a montage that can be created by using pencils, paints, chalks or pictures cut from magazines. The description can be written or spoken and can be recorded as a textual or audio-visual account. The purpose is for the community, based on their own interpretation, to describe their concerns. The role of the practitioner is to act as a guide to the community to think critically about their circumstances, their strengths (skills, knowledge), their access to external resources and their past ability to make decisions. The process may proceed as follows:

1   The individual/group is asked to discuss and produce a small drawing, audio-visual (video/DVD) or written description of their key concerns.
2   They are asked to clearly differentiate between each concern to avoid duplication or overlap.
3   The individual/group is asked to place these concerns into some kind of an order.
4   They are asked to rank their concerns, starting with the most important and ending with the least important. Concerns of equal important are placed together.
5   They are asked to comment on how they feel about each situation and should try to reach a consensus on the five most important concerns.

Ranking is a simple exercise in which issues can be 'unpacked' into their different elements so that they can be placed into a specific order and then further analysed. Ranking is also a way of prioritizing or categorizing issues that are important to the community. The order in which the issues are ranked is always determined by the community. The prioritized list can be scored, giving the highest score to the issue at the top of the list and the lowest score to the issue at the bottom. The practitioner discusses the reasons why one issue is scored higher than another in the list. When working with clients who are non-literate, pictures or drawings can be used instead of words to develop a ranked list. This simple technique provides information that can then be used to develop objectives to address concerns that can be accommodated into the programme (Laverack 2005: 48).

The programme defines the disease prevention issues to be addressed and in the context of chronic disease in Polynesian communities these include:

- reduce obesity/abdominal fat determined through body mass index;
- reduce hypertension;
- reduce dyslipidemia (high cholesterol);
- stop smoking.

The programming issue at stake then becomes how the 'disease prevention track' (defined by the outside agency) and the 'empowerment track' (defined by the community) can become linked during the progressive stages of the programme. The purpose of the programme is to achieve the disease prevention objectives and also to build community capacity to support the development of community empowerment. The financial, material, human and knowledge resources that are available through the programme are used to achieve this, in negotiation with the beneficiaries. As discussed in Chapter 2, community capacity-building is central to the process of community empowerment. Capacity-building involves the development of community skills, knowledge and competencies to address its concerns. In community empowerment these concerns explicitly include social and political change in favour of those trying to gain power.

The programme design may have to take into consideration the low level of skills and knowledge (capacity) that the community has at the beginning. Strategies can be developed as part of the design to build the necessary skills to increase the ability of the community to have more control over the management of the programme. The time necessary for a community to do this depends on the individual and collective capabilities of its members. Too short a programme timeframe runs the real risk of initiating community-level changes, only for the assistance to end before such changes have reached a satisfactory outcome.

The type of language and terminology used in the programme design can be an empowering experience for the intended beneficiaries. In practice, the advantage is often held by the one with the power-over (the practitioner) and the language that they choose to use can either strengthen or weaken the professional-client relationship. For example, the use of specialist language is often confusing to clients or to professionals not part of that professional sub-culture. This can contribute to their sense of powerlessness by emphasizing a lack of access to knowledge and the 'expert' power of the other person using the language. An empowering professional language is aware that no dis-course is value-free and is sensitive to the position and perceptions of clients. In particular, the practitioner should try to use a language that is open, respectful, non-coercive and uses simple technical terms that focus on the problems identified by the client. The practitioner uses positive words to build the power from within, for example, 'well done' or 'try again', and encourages the participation of the client. The practitioner also promotes the idea of a partnership with their client and encourages feedback and the sharing of ideas.

Setting programme objectives

The key question is: how are the programme (disease prevention) objectives and the empowerment objectives accommodated together in the design?

Objective-setting within chronic disease prevention is usually centred on a reduction in morbidity and mortality and on lifestyle management such as a change in specific health-related behaviours. Objective-setting for empowerment is centred on the level of control of the community over decisions regarding its health and its determinants. Parallel tracking gives the empowerment objectives an equal emphasis as the disease prevention objectives. The specific nature of the disease prevention objectives will vary according to the aims of the programme. The purpose of the parallel track is to provide empowerment objectives that complement the disease prevention objectives.

The empowerment objectives are based on community concerns. The role of the practitioner is to help the community members to write objectives that: are clear and achievable; are realistic and measurable; identify specific activities; sequence activities into an order to make the necessary improvements; assign individual roles and responsibilities to complete each activity; and set a realistic timeframe, including any significant benchmarks or targets.

In the example of the chronic disease prevention programme for a Polynesian community the empowerment objectives include:

- to assist the community to establish vegetable gardens in 20 locations in South and West Auckland before the end of 2008;
- to assist the community to establish five walking groups for Polynesian men and women in South and West Auckland before the end of 2008;
- to conduct 30 seminars on diabetes at community centres in South and West Auckland before the end of 2008.

The empowerment objectives need to be flexible as they are likely to change as the experiences of the community also change over time. This can be facilitated by the practitioner through dialogue and problem analysis to assist the community to narrow its focus towards more immediate and resolvable issues – for example, better access to exercise facilities to suit the needs of individual members.

The disease prevention objectives also need to be clear and achievable. For example, the programme will:

- reduce body mass index by 10 per cent in 50 per cent of the study population before the end of 2008;
- bring blood pressure readings into normal range for 50 per cent of the study population before the end of 2008;
- bring cholesterol levels into normal range for 50 per cent of the study population before the end of 2008;
- stop smoking in 50 per cent of the study population before the end of 2008.

Developing the strategic approach

The key question is: how does the strategic approach of the programme (disease prevention track) link with and strengthen the strategic approach for community empowerment?

This can be achieved by using approaches that are specifically designed to empower individuals to participate in groups, so that groups develop into community-based organizations centred on common interests and organizations strengthen their alliances and form partnerships. This is based on the continuum model of community empowerment (see Chapter 1).

The development of community organizations is crucial to allow small groups, and their individual members, to make the transition to a broader network of alliances. It is through these partnerships that organizations are able to gain greater support and resources to achieve a favourable outcome for their particular concerns. The key challenge in the strategic approach is how practitioners, and the agencies they represent, structure their work with the intention to assist individuals to organize collectively to form 'communities of interest' and partnerships. Linda Jones and Moyra Sidell (1997: 52–3), two respected commentators on health promotion, provide some useful steps for setting up and supporting partnerships and alliances – for example, helping the organization to identify its focus, aims and objectives, such as which health issue to address. The practitioner can also help by providing contacts to other alliances in the same area to avoid duplication of efforts, listing potential partners and helping the organization to set its own clear agenda, interests and goals. It is important that organizations meet regularly to discuss issues and review progress, and assign roles and responsibilities between their own members and partner organizations.

Programme management and implementation

The key question is: how does the implementation of the disease prevention track of the programme also systematically build community empowerment?

Health promotion programmes are typically managed by a practitioner or outside agent. The role of programme management has traditionally been to control or to have power over the process of planning, organizing and implementing the disease prevention objectives. The purpose has been to ensure success in terms of effectiveness (the extent to which objectives are achieved) and efficiency (the way in which the objectives are achieved compared to other means) (Ewles and Simnett 2003).

In bottom-up (empowerment) approaches the role of the programme management is to be sympathetic to stakeholder ownership and involvement and to make the programme an empowering experience for the community. This can be achieved by encouraging the community to take increasing responsibility for the management of the programme, for example by building skills and competencies to enable them to contribute to activities such as reporting, budgeting and evaluation. Table 4.1 provides specific examples of the type of training that can be included at each stage of a health promotion programme.

Table 4.1   Skills training in health promotion programmes

Programme phase	Skills training
Design	• Systematic review of literature • Analysis of epidemiological data • Identification of community needs • Appraisal of programme design
Objective-setting	• Developing SMART objectives • Logframe development
Strategic approach	• Strategies to empower individuals, groups and communities • Materials development • Health promotion models and theories • Interpersonal communication • Workshop facilitation • Conducting effective group meetings and public presentation
Programme management	• Fundraising • Budgeting • Conflict resolution • Resource procurement • Human resource management • Managing consultant inputs
Evaluation	• Participatory rural appraisal techniques • Qualitative research methods • Quantitative research methods • Visual representation

Another way of developing skills is to involve clients in short-term tasks that are realistic and achievable. To do this the practitioner can ask the community to set and achieve short-term goals. This is important because short-term successes can help to motivate people toward the achievement of long-term objectives. Progress should be periodically reviewed with the community to reflect on successes and failures (Laverack 2005). In the example of the chronic disease prevention programme for the Polynesian community this could include setting up a demonstration garden and the provision of skills training to encourage others to start their own vegetable garden. It could also include starting monthly walking groups before organizing more regular weekly groups.

Programme managers should increasingly give control to the community for the responsibilities of implementation. This requires the programme design to have a strategy for systematically developing the competencies, skills and capacities of the community such that it will have sufficient ability and confidence to maintain its strength and vitality.

Evaluation

The key question is: how does the evaluation of the programme outcomes also include empowerment?

The final stage of parallel tracking is the evaluation of both the programme (disease prevention) and the empowerment outcomes. Community empowerment can be a long process and if measured solely as an outcome its achievements can be lost during the relatively limited timeframe of top-down programming. The evaluation of changes in the course of a dynamic process of empowerment is therefore preferable to any particular outcome.

To continue with the example of a chronic disease prevention programme for a Polynesian community in Auckland, the evaluation of the empowerment outcomes set against the objectives includes:

- the number of active vegetable gardens that were established through the programme;
- the number of active walking groups for men and women established through the programme;
- the number of seminars completed.

By also measuring community empowerment as a process, it is possible to monitor the interaction between capacities, skills and resources at the individual and organizational levels during the timeframe of a programme. The evaluation of the programme as an empowering experience for all stakeholders, in particular the community, is better judged in terms of how they themselves assess achievements, through a participatory self-assessment. At an individual level, people experience a more immediate psychological empowerment (power from within), such as an increase in self-esteem or confidence. However, an evaluation that uses a self-assessment has to be careful to avoid an individual focus. It is the collective action that is to be measured because this shows the ability of the community to organize and mobilize itself toward social and political change.

The approach discussed in the next chapter provides a systematic means to measure community empowerment as a process by using nine 'domains'. The approach uses qualitative statements or 'descriptors' to guide community members to make a measurement of each domain. The self-evaluation is strengthened by using a systematic and structured approach to assist the community to focus on the relevant areas of influence. In programmes with limited resources the advantage is that this will reduce the timeframe and resources required by providing a focus on the relevant and specific areas of the process of community empowerment.

Chapter 5 uses case study examples to illustrate the importance of the nine domains to health promotion. The chapter also describes a step-by-step approach for building empowered communities within health promotion programming, including strategic planning.

5 'Unpacking' community empowerment for strategic planning

This chapter discusses the key domains of empowerment that enable communities to better organize themselves, both socially and structurally, towards the goal of social and political change. Empowerment is achieved through strategic planning to improve each 'domain', where a need has been identified by the members of a community. This is termed the 'domains approach' and has been used to build empowered communities within health promotion programming in Asia, Africa and the Pacific. In practice the approach involves setting a baseline for community empowerment and then developing a series of strategies to strengthen each domain. The chapter discusses the application of the 'domains approach' and how it can be adapted by practitioners to suit their different circumstances in health promotion programming.

The domains of community empowerment

Several authors have attempted to identify the areas of influence on community empowerment (Gibbon 1999; Laverack 2001) and in Table 5.1 I summarize the work of three authors to identify the 'domains' of three similar concepts: community participation, community capacity and community development.

The domains of empowerment represent how communities can better organize and mobilize themselves towards collective action including the aspects of social interaction and networking in a community. For example, the existence of functional leadership, supported by established organizational structures, with the participation of its members who have demonstrated the ability to mobilize resources, would indicate a community which already has strong social support elements. There are at least nine 'domains' for community empowerment (Laverack 2001), as follows:

1 Improves participation.
2 Develops local leadership.
3 Builds empowering organizational structures.

Table 5.1 The domains of three community-based concepts

Community participation factors (Rifkin et al. 1988)	Community capacity dimensions (Goodman et al. 1998)	Community development components (Labonte 1998)
	Participation	Participation
Leadership	Leadership	
Organization	Sense of community, its history and values	Community organization
Resource mobilization	Resources	Resource mobilization
Needs assessment		Priorities set using some form of analysis and targeted
	Critical reflection	Sharing of knowledge
	Social and interorganizational networks	Community as identity and locality
		Mediation skills
Management programme		Role of an outside agent
	Skills	Equitable relationships between community and agents
	Community power	Power dynamics

4 Increases problem assessment capacities.
5 Enhances the ability of the community to 'ask why' (critical awareness).
6 Improves resource mobilization.
7 Strengthens links to other organizations and people.
8 Creates an equitable relationship with outside agents.
9 Increases control over programme management.

Next is an interpretation of each domain. Case study examples of how to use the domains approach for building community empowerment are provided in Chapters 7 and 8.

Improves participation

Participation is basic to community empowerment. It describes the involvement of individuals in groups and in 'communities of interest' that share and have the capacity to begin to address their needs. In the context of health programming, community participation can be defined as:

> the process by which members of the community, either individually or collectively and with varying degrees of commitment: develop the capability to assume greater responsibility for assessing their health needs and problems; plan and then act to implement their solutions; create and maintain organizations in support of these efforts; and evaluate the effects and bring about necessary adjustments in goals and programmes on an on-going basis.
>
> (Zakus and Lysack 1998: 2)

This definition also encompasses many of the characteristics of an empowered community, essentially allowing people to become involved in activities which influence their lives and health. However, while individuals are able to influence the direction and implementation of a programme through their participation, this alone does not constitute community empowerment. For participation to be empowering it must not only involve the development of skills and abilities but must also raise critical awareness to enable people to make more informed decisions and to take action.

In a westernized context, the difference between participation and empowerment therefore lies in whether people simply 'participate' or actually take part in social and political *action*. To illustrate this, Box 5.1 provides an example of the interpretation of participation in a health promotion programme in a Fijian context.

Box 5.1   Participation and health promotion in a traditional Fijian context

Participation was not interpreted by the respondents of one project in Fiji as having a role in the decisions concerning design, implementation and evaluation. Their interpretation was more closely associated with Sherry Arnstein's (1969) degrees of tokenism (informing, consultation and placation). This may have been because their experience of programmes was limited to top-down approaches in which their input in decision-making were not required. However, it was also closely related to their own social structure in which every person has a predetermined role or responsibility. Katz (1993) points out that Fijian life is organized hierarchically, a system that permeates all aspects of life and can exclude many individuals from taking part in the decision-making process. Lewaravu (1986) further points out that the level of participation of each community member is differentiated by their traditional roles and tasks and it is the senior members of the community who take part in decision-making while the majority of people would only be involved in ceremonies or in activities such as food preparation.

Develops local leadership

Participation and leadership are closely connected because, just as leaders require a strong participant base, participation requires the direction and structure of strong leadership. Participation without a formal leader who takes responsibility for getting things done, deals with conflict and provides a direction for the group can often lead to disorganization (Goodman *et al.* 1998).

The structure of community leadership, which may be historically or culturally determined, can exclude marginalized groups and represent only the elite. Marginalization is a process by which an individual or a group of individuals are denied access to, or positions of, power – for example, economic and political influence – within a society (Marshall 1998). Certain groups within a community may not support the aim of a programme or local leaders may be in conflict with one another. Their inclusion can create dysfunction in the planning and implementation of the programme and make it more difficult to achieve the objectives. To exclude certain individuals and groups is undemocratic and does not fit within the ethos of empowerment that encourages community participation.

Karina Constantino-David (1995), a writer in community development, discusses the experiences of community organizing in the Philippines and the success of utilizing local leaders or 'organic organizers'. Competent leaders were developed by civil society organizations among poor people who offered a more insightful understanding of the community problems and culture. However, it was found that a lack of skills training and previous management experience among these people created limitations in their role as leaders. Leadership style and skills can therefore influence the way in which groups and communities develop and in turn this can influence empowerment.

Examples of leadership skills that can be enhanced through interventions in a health promotion programme context include:

- an empowerment style of leadership which encourages and supports the ideas and planning efforts of the community, using democratic decision-making processes and the sharing of information;
- collecting and analysing data; evaluating community initiatives; facilitation; and problem-solving;
- conflict resolution;

- the ability to connect to other leaders and organizations to gain resources and establish partnerships (Kumpfer 1993).

Builds empowering organizational structures

Organizational structures in a community include committees, faith groups, social and sports clubs and women's associations. These are the organizational elements which represent the ways in which people come together in order to address their concerns. They are also the way in which people come together to socialize – for example, to organize sporting and cultural events and to observe traditional customs and rituals. In this way the organizational structures help community members to interact and to connect. In a programme context it is also the way in which people come together to identify their problems, to find solutions to their problems and to plan for action to resolve their problems. The existence of, and the level at which, these organizations function is crucial to community empowerment. When existing organizational structures are not present, outside agencies have themselves established groups to address the programme concerns. However, the establishment of a new organizational structure such as a village health committee is insufficient to guarantee that it will be functional or that the community will organize itself. There must be a sense of community cohesion among its members. This is often characterized by a concern for community issues, a sense of connection to the people (family, friendships) and feelings of belonging manifested through customs, place, rituals and traditions.

The characteristics of a functional community organization have been found to include a membership of elected representatives that meet and participate on a regular basis. The members have an agreed membership structure (chairperson, secretary, core members etc.) that keeps records such as previous meetings and financial accounts. A functional community organization is also able to identify and resolve conflict quickly and its members are able to identify the 'problems' of, and the resources available to, their 'interest group' (Jones and Laverack 2003).

Increases problem assessment capacities

Problem assessment is most empowering when the identification of problems, solutions to the problems and actions to resolve the problems are carried out by the community. However, this fundamental principle continues to be a major shortcoming of many health promotion programmes. Practitioners must accept that the success of a programme depends to a great extent on the commitment and involvement of the intended beneficiaries. People are much more likely to be committed if they have a sense of ownership in regard to the problems and solutions being addressed by the programme. This is the case even if the problems being addressed are not those identified by the outside agent.

Outside agents obviously do often have new and useful information to offer, for example the latest information on how to prevent cancer. The point is that this information should not be imposed over the expressed needs and concerns that reside among community members. The best approach is to use a 'facilitated dialogue' between the community and the outside agents to allow the knowledge and priorities of both to decide an appropriate direction for the programme. Problem assessment undertaken by community members can also strengthen their role in the design of the programme. Programmes that do not address community concerns and that do not involve the community in the process of problem assessment usually do not achieve their purpose (Laverack 2004).

Enhances the ability of the community to 'ask why'

Generally small groups focus inwards on the needs of their members but as they develop into community organizations they must be able to broaden outwards to the environment that creates those needs in the first place. Asking 'why' is the ability of the community to be able to critically assess the underlying causes of their powerlessness. It is also the ability of the community to be able to develop strategies to bring about personal, social and political change based on an understanding of their own circumstances. Asking 'why' can be described as 'the ability to reflect on the assumptions underlying our and others' ideas and actions and to contemplate alternative ways of living' (Goodman et al. 1998: 272).

Fundamentally, 'asking why' is a process of discussion, reflection and collective action that is also called 'critical reflection', 'critical thinking' and 'critical consciousness'. The key term here is 'critical', where community members take a long, hard and analytical look at their situation and determine the social, political and economic reasons for their powerlessness. It has been described as a process of emancipation through learning or education, originally developed by the educationalist Paulo Freire in literacy programmes for slum dwellers in Brazil. People become the subjects of their own learning, involving critical reflection and an analysis of personal circumstances. This is achieved through group dialogue to share ideas and experiences and to promote critical thinking by posing problems to allow people to uncover the root causes of the unequal distribution of power. Once they are critically aware the group can start to plan actions to change the underlying political, economic and other circumstances that influence their lives.

Improves resource mobilization

The ability of a community to mobilize resources from within and to negotiate resources from beyond itself is an indication of a high degree of skill and organization. Goodman *et al.* (1998) discuss resources in terms of 'traditional capital', such as property and money, and 'social capital', which includes a sense of trust and the ability to cooperate with one another and with other communities. That communities possess both traditional and social capital is sometimes ignored by outside agents who bring with them the perceived necessary resources for the programme.

The outside agents may be expected to provide assistance to mobilize resources at the beginning of a programme but control over these must be increasingly carried out by the community, otherwise a paternalistic relationship can develop. Resources that health promoters might expect to mobilize from a community are traditionally based on voluntary labour (participation), materials, local knowledge and implementation insights, as well as some small financial contribution. There are paradoxically empowering reasons for expecting some financial, as well as human, resource contributions from the community. A community health promotion granting programme in Canada, for example, required some evidence of financial support from community proponents, which was to be matched by the funding agency at a 3:1 or greater basis. The reasoning was that if the community failed to mobilize any financial resources, the issues being proposed may not have strong community support and may reflect the interests only of the few persons making the programme proposal (Labonte 1996).

Strengthens links to other organizations and people

Links with other people and organizations include partnerships, coalitions and health alliances. Partnerships demonstrate the ability of the community to develop relationships with different groups or organizations based on recognition of overlapping or mutual interests, and interpersonal and interorganizational respect. They also demonstrate the ability to network, collaborate, cooperate and to develop relationships that promote a heightened interdependency among community members. Partnerships may involve an exchange of services, pursuit of a joint venture based on a shared goal or an advocacy initiative to change public or private policies.

A community-based coalition can be defined as 'a group of individuals representing diverse organisations, factions, or constituencies within the community who agree to work together to achieve a common goal' (Butterfoss *et al.* 1996: 66). Unlike partnerships, coalitions represent a diversity of views on a common issue and member groups have to learn to set aside differences and deal with internal conflicts. The outputs of links with other organizations and individuals may include proposals, recruitment of new members and the generation of resources resulting in improvements for the majority of the people in the community.

Health alliances can be described as cooperation and collaboration to create a partnership between organizations and individuals to enable people to increase control over, and to improve, their health. A health alliance is a collaboration that goes beyond health care and through the collective efforts of its members attempts to bring about social, political and environmental change to positively affect health (Jones *et al.* 2002).

Partnerships, coalitions and health alliances have become a popular theme within health promotion and are seen to be a two-way process incorporating both top-down and bottom-up principles of programming. It is implicit that the process is fully participatory and that government organizations do not merely consult or engage with people and the 'community'. People are involved in the decision-making processes of the programme, which has the aim of being an empowering experience.

Creates an equitable relationship with outside agents

Outside agents are practitioners, government employees, funding agencies, the representatives of agencies or organizations that do not form part of the community but are working with them to effect change. In a programme context the main role of the outside agent should be to link the community to resources or to assist the community to mobilize and organize itself to gain power. This can be especially important at the beginning of a programme when the process of community empowerment may be slow to start and the capacity of the community has to be built with the help of an outside agent.

The role of the outside agent is essentially one of the transformation of power over the control of decisions and resources, to allow clients to gain more control by discovering their own power from within.

The qualities of an empowering relationship in a programme context include:

- fostering the support of community and political leaders, including the involvement of marginalized groups;
- helping to negotiate new partnerships with other organizations;
- facilitating capacity-building through activities such as skills training and conflict management;
- developing specific skill areas such as self-evaluation.

The role of the outside agent as an evaluator is particularly important because they help to 'construct a shared vision of the past and future, provide judgements of project accomplishments, mediate stakeholder issues, build commitment to project objectives, and facilitate a consensus' (Thompson 1990: 379).

However, the role of the outside agent as an evaluator is somewhat contested in the literature. Cracknell (1996: 32) points out that there has been a shift in the role of the evaluator from 'that of disinterested observer to that of moderator ... negotiator ... [and] agents of change'. Other roles are as facilitator, enabler, coach and guide. It is difficult for many outside agents to be a neutral and detached observer of a programme when they often have so much invested in its success. While the outside agent is expected to make objective judgements about the quality and outcome of the programme, it should also be an empowering experience for the community. To facilitate this, the outside agent should ensure that community members are actively involved in the design and implementation of the evaluation, for example by using participatory techniques or self-assessment based on the knowledge and experience of community members.

Increases control over programme management

The role of the outside agent and programme management are closely linked and sometimes communities decide to combine these two domains for the purpose of assessment. At the heart of management is who controls the way in which the programme is designed, implemented, managed and evaluated.

Karina Constantino-David (1995) argues that the priorities of outside agents have shifted towards the expectation for better programme management, including financial systems. As programme management becomes more sophisticated the outside agents are less willing to transfer responsibility and skills to the community, which is perceived as having poor skills. Programme management that empowers the community includes control by the community members over all the decisions in regard to the programme. To do this the community must first have a sense of ownership of the programme, which in turn must address their needs and concerns. The role of the outside agent is to increasingly transform power relationships by transferring responsibility to the community through a systematic process of capacity-building.

Strategic planning for community empowerment

As discussed in Chapter 4, top-down programming is predominately used in health promotion and it is therefore the outside agent who identifies the issue to be addressed and who controls the implementation and evaluation. Plainly put, the programme is externally imposed and paternalistic. However, by using the domains approach it becomes easier for practitioners to engage with and help to empower communities. It is the beneficiaries who also identify concerns, who have increasing control of the programme and are able to develop strategies to address their concerns. The domains approach gives the practitioner a more precise way of developing strategies to build community empowerment. The key question practitioners need to ask themselves is: how has the programme, from its planning through its implementation, through its evaluation, intentionally sought to enhance community empowerment in each domain? (Laverack 2004).

The domains approach does not therefore start with a blank slate onto which people are expected to project their immediate concerns. The approach is participatory and has clear roles and responsibilities for all participants. In practical terms this allows the different participants of a programme to express their views, share their experiences and challenge existing values and beliefs. Different participants may have different opinions and the approach allows individuals to participate in an equal relationship that facilitates the involvement of each member through discussion and interaction with one another.

The domains approach is implemented in four steps (Laverack 2003):

1   Preparation, including the development of a culturally appropriate definition for empowerment.
2   Setting a baseline for each domain.
3   Strategic planning and the assessment of resources.
4   Evaluation and visual representation.

Step 1: preparation

It is important to use interpretations of power and empowerment that are relevant and important to the participants, set within their cultural context. Westernized concepts of power and empowerment can have different interpretations to those in social settings in non-westernized countries. The idea is to use terms that have been identified and defined by the clients themselves to provide a mutual understanding of the programme in which they are involved and toward which they are expected to contribute. A working definition of power and empowerment is developed through the use of simple qualitative methods. I provide an example of how this definition was developed in a Fijian context in Box 5.2.

The nine empowerment domains, although comprehensive, may exclude areas of influence that are relevant to community members. It is important to carry out a period of discussion prior to Step 2 to adapt the meaning of each domain in order to meet the requirements of the cultural context. The domains approach is flexible in that it allows the selected domains to be changed, if necessary, during the programme.

> **Box 5.2** Developing a working definition of empowerment in Fiji
>
> In Fiji, the use of simple qualitative techniques has been shown to identify the key terms in regard to power and empowerment. Unstructured interviews were first used to identify the headings for power-over, or *lewa*, power from within and power-with, or *kaukauwa*. Then, through semi-structured interviews the term *lewa* was further identified to refer to 'chiefly *lewa*', the control of the village chief and the power-over bestowed at work or in the home. The term *kaukauwa* is the closest concept in a Fijian context to empowerment. It refers to community strength and unity which can be developed and assisted by its members and can be used to describe the right a person has to do something. Chiefly, *lewa* is a state, a status which is bestowed by birthright or by others in an accepted way and is inter-dependent on the strength or *kaukauwa* of the community. It is in the interests of the person with the chiefly *lewa* and the members of the community to maintain and increase the *kaukauwa*. The relationship is reciprocal and in this way the *lewa* and *kaukauwa* play an important role in the unity and strength of the community. The *kaukauwa* may be a mechanism by which the members of a community manage the authority delegated to them by the person with the *lewa*. It may also be a mechanism used when the community decides to resist and challenge this au-thority. Although the two terms provide a common understanding this can depend on how they are used. For example, the term *kaukauwa* in the form *veivakakau-kauwataki*, suggests action and a process rather than just a concept and would be a more useful term to use in a programme context (Laverack 2005: 90).

Step 2: setting a baseline for each domain

The approach is usually conducted in a 'workshop'-style setting. A workshop is a westernized term which is defined here as a group meeting to provide a convenient way for different people to come together and exchange ideas and experiences, and to learn about techniques, models and skills. The focus of the workshop is on participatory activities involving discussion and problem-solving exercises towards practical, action-orientated outcomes based on the consensus of its members. The workshop design has to be flexible and needs to consider some basic elements such as the homogeneity of the group, its dynamics, size and the timeframe for the exercises. It typically takes one day to complete the baseline assessment (Step 2) and one day to complete the strategic plan (Step 3). The participants of the workshop are representatives of a 'community' or the individual representatives of groups that share the same interests and needs. However, it is unlikely that all members of a community are able to take part in a workshop, which can usually only accommodate 15–20 people. This raises the issue, discussed in Chapter 2, of who should re-present the community.

Setting the baseline

The community representatives first make an assessment of each domain. To do this they are provided with five statements for each empowerment domain, each written on a separate sheet of paper. The five statements represent a description of the various levels of empowerment related to that domain. Taking one domain at a time, the participants are asked to select the statement which most closely describes the present situation in their community. The statements are not numbered or marked in any way and each is read out loud by the participants to encourage group discussion. The descriptions may be amended by the participants or a new description may be provided to describe the situation for a particular domain. In this way the participants make their own assessment for each domain by comparing their experiences and opinions.

Recording the reasons why

Recording the reasons why the assessment has been made for each domain is important so that this information can be taken into account during subsequent assessments. It also provides some defensible or empirically observable criteria for the selection. This overcomes one of the weaknesses in the use of qualitative statements, that of reliability over time or across different participants making the assessment (Uphoff 1991). The justification needs to include verifiable examples of the actual experiences of the participants taken from their community to illustrate in more detail the reasoning behind the selection of the statement.

The five statements in Figure 5.1 represent short scenarios of a range of potentially empowering situations in regard to the domain 'increases problem assessment capacities'. The selection of one statement represented an independent assessment, reached by consensus and based on the experiences and knowledge of all the participants.

Table 5.2 provides generic statements for each domain which can be adapted to different cultural contexts. The table also shows the rating for each statement. This is used as a record by the facilitators of the workshop to determine a score once the selection has been completed by the participants. This rating is not shared with the participants prior to the assessment, to avoid the introduction of bias.

NA I TIKOTIKO E SEGA KINA NA KILA KEI NA VAKAVAKARAU ME QARAVI KINA NA VAKADIDIKE
Community lacks skills and awareness to carry out an assessment

E SEGA NI VAKADIKEVI NA LEQA E NA VEI TIKOTIKO
No problem assessment undertaken by the community

NA I TIKOTIKO E TIKO KINA NA KILA. NA LEQA KEI NA I TUVATUVA NI KA ME VAKAYACORI KA RA VAKARAITAKA MAI NA LEWE NI I TIKOTIKO.
E SEGA NI RA VAKAITAVI KINA NA I SOQOSOQO LALAI ESO E NA I TIKOTIKO
Community has skills. Problems and priorities identified by the community. Did not involve participation of all sectors of the community

NA LEQA , NAVEIKA E SA VAKAYACORI, KEI NA KEDRA I WALI E SA VAKATAKILAI MAI E NA I TIKOTIKO. E VAKYACORI NA VAKADIDIKE ME VAKAQAQACOTAKI KINA NA I TUVATUVA NI I TIKOTIKO
Community identified problems, solutions and actions. Assessment used to strengthen community planning

ME TOSO TIKO GA NA KENA VAKAQARAI NA LEQA, NA KENA I WALI KEI NA VEIKA E SA VAKAYACORI ENA I TIKOTIKO
Community continues to identify and is the owner of problems, solutions and actions

Figure 5.1   Statements used for 'increases problem assessment capacities' in Fiji
Source: Laverack (1999: 169)

Table 5.2 The generic statements for each domain and ranking

Domain	1	2	3	4	5
Community participation	Not all community members and groups are participating in community activities and meetings (e.g. women, youth, men)	Community members are attending meetings but not involved in discussion and helping	Community members involved in discussions but not in decisions on planning and implementation. Limited to activities such as voluntary labour and financial donations	Community members involved in decisions on planning and implementation. Mechanism exists to share information between members	Participation in decision-making has been maintained. Community members involved in activities outside the community
Problem assessment capacities	No problem assessment undertaken by the community	Community lacks skills and awareness to carry out an assessment	Community has skills. Problems and priorities identified by the community. Did not involve participation of all sectors of the community	Community identified problems, solutions and actions. Assessment used to strengthen community planning	Community continues to identify and is the owner of problems, solutions and actions
Local leadership	Some community organizations without a leader	Leaders exist for all community organizations. Some organizations	Community organizations functioning under leaders. Some Organizations do not	Leaders are taking initiative with support from their organizations.	Leaders taking full initiative. Organizations in full support. Leaders work with outside

Domain	1	2	3	4	5
		not functioning under their leaders	have the support of leaders outside the community	Leaders require skills training	groups to gain resources
Organizational structures	Community has no organizational structures such as committees	Organizations have been established by the community but are not active	More than one organization active. Organizations have mechanism to allow members to provide meaningful participation	Many organizations have established links with each other within the community	Organizations actively involved in and outside the community. Community committed to its own and to other organizations
Resource mobilization	Resources are not being mobilized by the community	Only rich and influential people mobilize resources raised by community. Community members are made to give resources	Community has increasingly supplied resources, but no collective decision about distribution. Resources raised have had limited benefits	Resources raised also used for activities outside the community. Discussion by community on distribution but not fairly distributed	Considerable resources raised and community decide on distribution. Resources fairly distributed
Links to others	None	Community has informal links with other organizations and people. Does not have a well-defined purpose	Community has agreed links but is not involved in community activities and development	Links interdependent, defined and involved in community development, based on mutual respect	Links generating resources, finances and recruiting new members. Decisions resulting in improvements for the community

Domain	1	2	3	4	5
Ability to 'ask why'	No group discussions held to ask why about community issues	Small group discussions are being held to ask why about community issues and to challenge received wisdom	Groups held to listen to community issues. These have the ability to reflect on assumptions underlying their ideas and actions. Are able to challenge received wisdom	Dialogue between community groups to identify solutions, self-test and analyse. Some experience of testing solutions	Community groups have ability to self-analyse and improve efforts over time. This is leading toward collective change
Programme management	By agent	By agent in discussion with community	By community supervised by agent. Decision-making mechanisms mutually agreed. Roles and responsibilities clearly defined. Community has not received skills training in programme management	By community in planning, policy and evaluation with limited assistance from agent. Developing sense of community ownership	Community self-manage independent of agent. Management is accountable.

Domain	1	2	3	4	5
Relationship with outside agent	Agents in control of policy, finances, resources and evaluation of the programme	Agents in control but discuss with community. No decision-making by community. Agent acting on behalf of agency to produce outputs	Agents and community make joint decisions. Role of agent mutually agreed	Community makes decisions with support from agents. Agent facilitates change by training and support	Agents facilitate change at request of community which makes the decisions. Agent acts on behalf of the community to build capacity

Source: Laverack (1999)

Step 3: strategic planning and the assessment of resources

The purpose of the baseline assessment in Step 2 is for community members to set a measurement for their own level of collective empowerment at that particular time. The information collected during the baseline assessment can then be used by the community to move forward to build their knowledge, skills and capacities toward gaining more power. This is a process of learning through strategic planning. The baseline assessment in itself is insufficient to empower the participants who must also have the ability to transform this information into individual and collective action. The purpose of the strategic planning is therefore to bring about positive actions in each of the domains where a need for improvement has been identified by the community. Three simple steps are used for strategic planning: a discussion on how to improve the present situation; the development of a strategy to improve upon the present situation; and the identification of any necessary resources for the implementation of the strategic plan.

How to improve the present situation

Following the baseline assessment of each domain the participants are asked how this situation can be improved in their community. If more than one statement has been selected the participants should consider how to improve each situation separately. The purpose is to identify the broader approaches that will improve the present situation and provide a pathway into a more detailed strategy. If the participants decide that the present situation does not require any improvement, no strategy will be developed for that particular domain.

Developing a strategy to improve the present situation

The participants are next asked to consider how, in practice, the present baseline assessment can be improved. The participants develop a more detailed strategy based on the broader approaches that have already been identified, for example by:

- identifying activities listed and broken into sub-components or activities in an appropriate series which will ultimately lead to an improvement;
- sequencing activities to ensure that they are sorted into the correct order to make an improvement;
- setting a realistic timeframe including any significant benchmarks or targets;
- assigning responsibilities to specific individuals to complete each activity within the specified timeframe.

An assessment of resources

The participants assess the internal and external resources that are necessary to improve the present situation. They typically identify internal resources such as commitment to the strategies developed, attendance at meetings and better interpersonal communication. The participants also identify external resources such as skills training and small financial grants. The request for external resources is typically modest and the participants firstly seek resources from within the community, recognizing that they often possess the necessary skills and knowledge to implement their own strategies.

Developing a framework for the strategy

The information obtained from the development of a strategic plan can be combined with the baseline assessment for each domain into a simple framework. The purpose is to provide a summary of the assessment and strategic plan. In Table 5.3 I provide an example of a completed framework for seven of the domains for the Naloto community in Fiji. The domains for 'programme management' and the 'role of the outside agent' were not included because the community had not yet established a partnership with an outside agency. The framework was used by the community to later attract funds to support a health promotion programme.

Down the left-hand column are listed the domains. The next two columns refer to the baseline assessment and the reasons why the assessment has been made. The framework can include the rating given to each assessment so that this can be discussed or visually represented. When the participants cannot agree upon the selection of one domain the rating is taken as the average value of the statements selected.

The next two columns of the framework refer to the development of a strategic plan for community empowerment (how to improve the present assessment) and a strategy for implementation to improve the assessment (where this is necessary). The participants most often identify approaches for the improvement of the present situation that are feasible to themselves. For example, in the Naloto community, they selected:

- increasing local leadership and management skills;
- regular meetings to improve the flow of information between the leaders and the community;
- developing a clear plan of action or directive that states roles and responsibilities.

The final column outlines the resources necessary to implement the strategy, for example, the Naloto community selected a year planner, human resources to conduct training, a venue to hold the training and funds to support transport to reach the training venue.

Table 5.3 The framework for assessment and strategic planning for the Naloto community in Fiji

Domain	Baseline assessment			Development of the strategy	
	Baseline assessment	Reasons why selected	How to improve	Implementation	Resources
Resource mobilization *Na kena vakayagataki na i yau bula*	Community has increasingly supplied resources but no collective decision about distribution. Resources raised have had limited benefits. Rating 3	People have given resources for planned activities but these were not carried out. Resources continue to be requested from the community	Considerable resources need to be raised by the community. Community should decide on the distribution which should be carried out fairly	A clear plan of action to include policy of accountability. Regular meetings. Provide feedback from meetings to community. Leadership and management training to set a good example	Year planner. Meeting place and small funds to hold meeting. Timeframe for meetings. Skills training for leaders
Participation *Vakaitavi/Cakacaka vata*	Not all community groups are participating in activities and meetings such as youth groups. Rating 1	There is a lack of knowledge skills, focus and interest in the community. Personal differences divide the community	Use traditional protocol, chiefly leadership and *matagali*. Have a clear directive on the course of action	Develop directive with timeframe, activities, responsibilities in follow-up meetings	Human resources to develop directive. Commitment to implement
Organizational structures	Organizations have been established by the community but they are not active.	A lack of leadership skills and commitment. Time constraints on	Skills training for leaders. Clarify role of leaders. Improve channels of	Training programme for leaders. Regular meetings by Tikina council.	Training support from outside agent. Funds or transportation for

Domain	Baseline assessment		How to improve	Development of the strategy	
	Baseline assessment	Reasons why selected		Implementation	Resources
Na tuvatuva I ni cakacaka se veiqaravi vei ira nai soqosoqo	Rating 2	outside leaders (health workers) to reach community	communication between leaders and community. Provide notice for time of meetings. Improve networking	Regular visits to meetings by leaders to discuss issues raised	leaders to reach community
Problem assessment *Vakadikevi ni leqa*	Community lacks the necessary skills and awareness to carry out its own problem assessment. Rating 2	History of petty theft in community. History of conflict within village groups and unable to reach consensus	Improve leadership skills. The delegation of tasks to every able-bodied man in the community	Training programme for leaders. Regular meetings by Tikina council. Regular visits to meetings by leaders to discuss issues raised	Training support from outside agent. Funds or transportation for leaders to reach community
Links with others *Na I sema ki na vei soqosoqo kei na lewe ne vanua*	Community has agreed links but not involved in activities and development. Rating 3	A lack of information and knowledge within the community about outside links	Improve the availability and flow of information. Improve the channels of communication between 'bottom and top' community to leaders	Training programme for leaders. Regular meetings by Tikina council. Regular visits to meetings by leaders to discuss issues raised	Training support from outside agent. Funds or transportation for leaders to reach community

Domain	Baseline assessment			Development of the strategy	
	Baseline assessment	Reasons why selected	How to improve	Implementation	Resources
Leadership *Veiliutaki*	Community organizations functioning under leaders *but* leaders require skills training. Rating 3.5	Have not received skills training A lack of role identification by leaders. Inadequate support for their needs as leaders	Skill training for leaders. Clarify role of leaders. Improve channels of communication between leaders and community. Improve networking	Training programme for leaders. Regular meetings by Tikina council. Regular visits to meetings by leaders to discuss issues raised	Training support from outside agent. Funds or transportation for leaders to reach community
Asking why *Na nodra vakatataro na lewe ni vanua va cava e vakavuna se baleta na cava?*	Small group discussions are being held to ask why about community issues and to challenge the received wisdom. Rating 2		Not necessary at this stage		

Source: Laverack (1999: 244)

In practice, the framework provides the basis for further discussion, planning and action by the participants. The participants can meet to further review the assessment and the strategies that they have developed. This process builds the knowledge, skills and confidence of the participants to take control of the issues influencing their lives, outlined in the framework.

The role of the practitioner is to facilitate the execution of the strategy by providing technical assistance and some of the resources identified as part of the framework. The practitioner also has a role to help share information received with the participants to maintain community support and promote accountability. The framework outlines what goals and activities have been set by the community over a specified timeframe and what support will be given by the practitioner. An important part of this process is the identification of specific roles and responsibilities among the participants to monitor the progress made toward achieving the strategy. Regular meetings between the community and the practitioner are also held to determine progress in achieving community empowerment through a strengthening of the domains. This can be aided by using an appropriate method of visual representation of the rating of each domain (see Chapter 6).

The goal is to encourage the community members to develop a sense of ownership in regard to the strategy that they have identified as being important to them. This commitment will inevitably ebb and flow and may not necessarily be in coordination with programme deadlines or targets. However, by agreeing a timeframe with the participants for implementation the practitioner can design the programme inputs and outputs to include the activities and resources identified in the framework. This is usually carried out over a six-month timeframe to implement several of the strategies identified for specific domains. The progress of achieving each strategy can then be evaluated at the end of each six-month period and this forms the basis for further discussion and planning.

It is not always possible to develop a detailed strategy of activities and sub-activities. In this situation it is important to hold follow-up meetings to further discuss the implementation of the strategies and to identify who will be responsible. It may not be feasible to implement the whole strategy and this can be carried out in stages using some of the domains within a realistic timeframe.

The domains approach is flexible and a strategic plan for community empowerment can be developed in various ways. For example, the participants can discuss the best way forward to improve each domain and a summary of the plan can be agreed upon and then documented. The community members can still participate in and make a contribution toward the programme with the advantage that this can be done much quicker – for example, during a community meeting – and with limited resources. Case study examples of how the domains approach has been used are provided in

Chapter 7 (in an issues-based approach) and Chapter 8 (in a community-based approach).

Step 4: evaluation and visual representation

The progress, or regression, of each domain can be measured and then visually represented as a part of programme evaluation using a spider-web configuration. This is discussed in detail in Chapter 6.

6 Evaluating community empowerment

The purpose of evaluation in a programme context

There is no real agreement about the overall purpose of evaluation in a health promotion programme context. However, it should address the concerns of the programme stakeholders who require information about its impact, operation, progress and achievements. Evaluation is an integral part of management (Usher 1995) with the purpose of providing inputs to ongoing activities and information for future design, effectiveness (have I met my targets?) and efficiency (the outputs in relation to the inputs). Evaluation also has a role in the accountability of programmes, usually to the outside agent who contributes to the funding (Rebien 1996).

In top-down programming, evaluation is used as an instrument of control through performance measurement. The aim is to improve performance in terms of achieving targets by providing feedback about the operational elements of the programme implementation. The evaluation typically uses predetermined indicators, toward which the primary stakeholders do not contribute, and is often implemented by an outside 'expert'. Bottom-up programming places the focus on the process toward participatory self-evaluation and away from conventional 'expert'-driven approaches. This means a fundamental shift in the power relationship between the outside agents and the beneficiaries of the programme, one where control over decisions about design and evaluation is more equitably distributed. A range of methodologies have been designed to assist communities to undertake self-assessments including participatory rural appraisal (PRA), participatory learning appraisal and participatory action research. Participatory evaluation aims to empower the participants involved in the process. In practice, this means actively involving people in the implementation of the evaluation and providing them with the means to make decisions to improve their lives and health.

An example of a participatory approach used to empower others is PRA, which became an increasingly popular 'tool' to assess and monitor improvements in the health and development of communities in the 1990s. It is not a clearly defined single technique but a collection of participatory approaches and methods to enable people to present, share and analyse information that they themselves have identified as being important. PRA has also been used for its potential to empower communities on the basis that it actively involves the marginalized, assesses their needs, builds capacities and includes them in the decision-making process. PRA can produce a large amount of information that is related to the physical and social elements of a programme but has been criticized (James 1995) for not addressing the underlying structural causes of powerlessness such as resource control. PRA does not always offer a means to the community to transform information into social and political action, a crucial stage in the process of community empowerment. This is important, otherwise the powerful dominate and exclude others, and expectations are raised and then disappointed by a lack of means to translate information into action. The process of evaluation merely becomes one of needs assessment and participation rather than an empowering experience.

Design considerations

Empowering approaches for evaluation redefine the role relationship between stakeholders. The role of the outside agent has been traditionally viewed as one of 'expert' or 'professional', one who judges merit or worth (Patton 1997). This role is changed in an empowering approach to one who facilitates, enables, coaches and guides other stakeholders (Fetterman *et al.* 1996). The evaluation itself becomes an empowering experience by building capacity, skills, competencies, the power from within of individuals and the power-with of practitioners. This can be illustrated in the idea of 'empowerment evaluation' which has gained prominence in the USA (see Box 6.1).

Box 6.1 Empowerment evaluation

'Empowerment evaluation' can be defined as the 'use of evaluation concepts, techniques, and findings to foster improvement and self-determination' (Fetterman *et al.* 1996: 4). To achieve this, the approach uses both qualitative and quantitative techniques in group activities as an ongoing process of internalized and institutionalized evaluation. The emphasis of the approach is very much on self-determination targeted at the disenfranchised in a world where power cannot be given but must be gained or taken by people. The steps of 'empowerment evaluation' are: (1) taking stock of the programme's weaknesses and strengths; (2) establishing goals for future improvement; (3) developing strategies to achieve the goals; and (4) determining the type of evidence required to document credible progress toward those goals. The role of the evaluator is one of facilitator rather than 'expert' (Fetterman *et al.* 1996).

Uphoff (1991) points out that there are at least four benefits to utilizing participatory self-evaluations over conventional assessments by an outside agent: self-educative; self-improving; enables stakeholders to monitor progress; and improves training. Participatory self-assessments motivate the stakeholders to identify and build on their strengths and to minimize their weaknesses through their own efforts. In a practical sense, self-evaluation is based on the experiences of the stakeholders which, as far as possible, is not influenced by the methodology or has not been biased by the evaluator. The evaluator and the procedures they use attempt to capture aspects of the social world through observing and recounting the lived experiences of people. Consequently, these types of strategies have been criticized for being subjective, impressionistic, idiosyncratic and biased (Uphoff 1991).

To some extent the evaluator's presence will influence the findings of the evaluation. Even at its most basic, having an evaluator observing actions may stimulate modifications in behaviour or action, or encourage introspection or self-questioning among those participating (Mays and Pope 1995). The participants themselves may also be a source of bias. Robson (1993) provides an example of 'subject bias' when pupils who seek to please their teacher, knowing the importance or reward they will receive from a good result or the result desired by the teacher, will change their behaviour or make a stronger effort at a test.

Guba and Lincoln (1989: 233–43) suggest the following considerations for the dependability, transferability and confirmability of a participatory evaluation. These are useful principles that can be applied in the design of empowerment approaches to maintain rigour and credibility.

- Techniques that use thick descriptive data from qualitative interviews, observation and detailed field notes.
- Verification of data with stakeholders, for example, to cross-check cultural interpretations.
- Triangulation using different methods and data sources.
- Audit trail of the design through a clear documentation from data to conclusions reached.
- Verification of interpretations by other evaluators through inter-observer agreement.
- 'Hard' questioning of findings by peers through a work-in-progress critique.
- Critical self-reflection on meanings of the findings and relevance to stakeholders.
- An emphasis in the findings on what is useful.

Selecting an appropriate paradigm

There are a number of different models that can be considered for the measurement of community empowerment, for example, critical theory which holds that knowledge must be situated historically and cannot be a matter of universal or timeless abstract principles. Two ideal types of paradigm that are relevant to the selection of an appropriate approach for the measurement of community empowerment are positivist and constructivist (Guba 1990). A paradigm can be defined as a world view that is composed of multiple belief categories, principal among them being their ontological, epistemological and methodological assumptions. Ontological assumptions are about the way in which the world is, the nature of reality. Epistemological assumptions are about what we can know about that reality. Methodological assumptions are about how we come to know that reality and the strategies we employ in order to discover the way in which the world functions.

The 'conventional' paradigm is typified as the positivist approach. Its ontology consists of a belief in a single reality, independent of any observer, and a belief that universal truths independent of time and place exist and can be discovered. Its epistemology consists of a belief that the evaluator can and should investigate a phenomenon in a way that is uncluttered by values and biases. The methodology of the conventional paradigm favours experimental designs to test hypotheses and is concerned with prediction through proof or certainty and with singular measures of reality and truth. Applications of this paradigm can be seen in medicine, and in approaches used in health promotion such as epidemiology and in top-down programming (Labonte and Robertson 1996).

The constructivist approach provides a wider framework in which 'truth' and 'fact' are recognized as having subjective dimensions. What emerges from this process is an agenda for negotiation based on the claims and issues raised during dialogue between the evaluator and those they are involved with in the evaluation. Its ontology is relativist, meaning that realities are socially constructed. Realities are local and specific, dependent on their form and content and on the persons who hold them. Its epistemology recognizes the evaluator as part of the reality that is being evaluated and the findings as a creation of the enquiry process. The findings are literally the creation of the process of interaction between the enquirer and enquired. Its methodology focuses on people's experiences as being located in a particular socio-historical context. Individual constructions are elicited, refined, compared and contrasted with the aim of generating one or more constructions on which there is substantial consensus. In the constructivist paradigm truth is not absolute, but rather is understood as the best informed and most sophisticated truth we might construct at any given moment. This paradigm seeks to know by understanding how and what people experience within their own context, and its application can be seen in community development and in bottom-up programming (Labonte and Robertson 1996).

The concept of empowerment is concerned with the experiences, opinions and knowledge of people. It is a construction of individual and collective local beliefs and truths. Empowerment can have a different meaning to different people in the same programme and the selection of an appropriate paradigm should therefore account for different subjective experiences and allow these to be accessed (Rappaport 1985). Labonte and Robertson (1996) argue that much of the debate in regard to health promotion has been around the issues of methods, in particular 'hard' quantitative versus 'soft' qualitative, rather than around methodology. Qualitative methods can be used in positivist ways just as quantitative methods can be used by constructionists. However, although it is fairly easy to triangulate different methods, it is quite another matter to triangulate different ontological and epistemological approaches. It is the ontological and epistemological differences which are fundamental between the two main paradigms, constructivism and positivism (Guba 1990). The challenge in the selection of an appropriate paradigm is about the epistemological stance and the relationships of power embedded within the process of evaluation.

A constructivist paradigm can accommodate both qualitative and quantitative methods and the ontological and epistemological assumptions are better suited to the evaluation of empowerment. These assumptions allow the experiences and knowledge of those being evaluated to be taken into account. Health promotion has tended to operate from within a positivist paradigm, especially those programmes which have used a top-down approach. To a much lesser extent has health promotion operated within a constructivist paradigm when using bottom-up and empowerment approaches (Labonte and Robertson 1996).

Ethical and practical considerations

There are several underlying ethical and practical considerations that can help to guide the practitioner in developing an evaluation approach for community empowerment:

- the approach is equitable and inclusive to allow all members of the community to express their views, share their experiences and challenge existing values and beliefs;
- the approach respects ethnic diversity and recognizes that different participants may have different opinions;
- the approach allows individuals to participate in an equal relationship with one another and with the practitioner, who facilitates the involvement of each member through discussion and interaction;
- the approach establishes relationships, builds trust and partnerships of people working together to address local concerns;

- the approach facilitates a process of capacity-building of the community members towards greater control over their own evaluation;
- the approach is an empowering experience in that it provides a means to translate the information gained into individual and collective decision-making actions;
- the approach develops a long-term commitment for empowerment from both the community and from the outside agency.

At an organizational level it is necessary to develop an institutional and management strategy that considers these principles for the evaluation of community empowerment. This occurs from the top tiers of policy and planning 'down' to the people working at the interface with the community. The outside agencies build their organizational capacity and strengthen management practices, internal structures and the commitment to pursue appropriate evaluation approaches. This is reflected in the discourse of the policy of the agency: the language, rhetoric, values and ideology that it uses, all of which are instrumental in facilitating the processes of capacity-building and empowerment.

As a further guide to agencies working with communities, the organizational principles for evaluation should include:

- The values of the agency (e.g. does it perceive that it is important to involve the community in identifying community health issues and developing programmes? Does it recognize that partnering and collaborating with other groups or community-based organizations is important?).
- The intent of the agency (e.g. what is the best way to establish its position and select strategies for community action? Are authoritative approaches or cooperative approaches more appropriate?).
- The operations of the agency (e.g. is it already working with the community around specific programmes or issues? How? Are there existing collaborations with other institutions or agencies? Are community leaders or representatives already involved in decision-making related to programme evaluation?).
- The resources and expertise available to support an evaluation (e.g. what mechanisms are in place to ensure that relevant data on community needs will be used? What financial resources will be required? Which staff are most skilled or already have strong ties to the community?) (adapted from CDC/ATSDR 1997).

Ronald Labonte and Ann Robertson (1996), two prominent Canadian health promoters, and Yoland Wadsworth and Maggie McGuiness (1992), two prominent Australian commentators, raise further points in regard to the ethical commitments required from those involved in evaluating community empowerment:

- a fundamental respect for all parties as equal, a determination to seek their perceptions and an opportunity for all to discuss and interpret the findings in order to reach a consensus on the best explanation;
- to negotiate an equitable relationship between the evaluator and those persons or groups with whom they are working, central to this being flexibility in the power relationship between professionals and their 'clients';
- a commitment to understanding that different parties have different values, concerns and meanings and that these are all equally important.

These commitments provide the basis for the design characteristics of an evaluation methodology: an approach which is participatory and empowering, allows a self-assessment and is appropriate within a programme context. The key characteristics for the evaluation of community empowerment are summarized in Box 6.2.

Box 6.2 Key characteristics for the evaluation of community empowerment

Design

- Applies principles of rigour that are technically sound, theoretically underpinned and field-tested.
- Uses an appropriate method.
- Addresses programme effectiveness and efficiency.
- Addresses programme achievements and inputs.
- Addresses ethical concerns.

Stakeholder needs

- Clearly defines the roles and responsibilities of all stakeholders.
- Use participatory, self-evaluation approaches.
- Information provided can be interpreted by all stakeholders.

Outcomes

- Provides information that is accurate and feasible.
- Is empowering such that the stakeholders can use the information to make decisions and take action.
- Findings use a mix of interpretation (e.g. textual and visual).

Methodological considerations

The development of an evaluation 'tool' or approach to measure community empowerment raises several methodological considerations in a health promotion programme context.

Defining and measuring an inclusive community

No community is homogenous and this makes the inclusion of all community members or their representatives difficult. Georgia Bell-Woodward *et al.* (2005) found that a review of the history of the initiative, and encouragement of respondents to 'visualize what an outsider would see' were helpful. Bell-Woodard *et al.* raise the issue of how to motivate the community to participate in the measurement of community empowerment. Only 5 of the 14 community representatives responded to their short written survey. This was indicative of their level of participation at the time the survey was done, and the energy available from the initiative's staff to involve them.

Creation of valid knowledge from diverse perspectives and participation

Validity in assessments, such as using qualitative statements, can be problematic for at least three reasons: to an extent, people are assessing their own work; perceptions are prone to recall bias; and ratings in a group setting may be influenced by the dynamics of the group. Bell-Woodward *et al.* found that these validity concerns were partly met by an emphasis on people providing reasons and examples for their ratings, prefacing the assessments with a brief recounting of the history of the initiative and ensuring that individuals made their assessments prior to sharing them in the group. Laverack (1999) found that his participants quickly became aware of the link between each qualitative statement when making a rating. This led to a shift in the overall ranking assessment towards the higher range between 'satisfactory' and 'most satisfactory'. This was a 'demand response' bias, inherent in the use of undisguised progressive (from least to most) rating scales. In addition to the design features of the methodology, this behaviour may be explained by both the influence of the practitioner and by bias introduced by the participants. In order to deal with this type of bias it is essential to make sure that the evaluation is rigorous and that the evaluator's unavoidable sympathies are made open as a part of the account to try and avoid the distortions that bias may introduce into the evaluation.

The problematic use of rating scales to measure empowerment

A rating scale is a series of items that measures a single variable or domain. The items are placed in a single index or continuum and provide a range of points which represent a measure from, for example, the least to the most. This range can be classified numerically or by using descriptions of each point on the continuum (Litwin 1995).

A structured approach to assessment has been utilized by a number of authors who have developed rating scales to provide a more systematic methodology for community participation (Shrimpton 1995; Balcazar and Suarez-Balcazar 1996) and community competence (Eng and Parker 1994). Uphoff (1991) developed a self-evaluation methodology for 'people's participation' programmes in developing countries. The methodology uses the selection from a set of questions which are relevant to the needs of the programme, such as the maintenance of equipment or the provision of infrastructure. The methodology then develops an assessment based on these questions. Uphoff uses questions arranged into four alternatives ranging from an ideal to an unacceptable situation. Each alternative is given a score ranging from 0 to 3. Kirsten Havemann (2006) developed a tool for the visualization and calculation of an overall effectiveness score of participation and empowerment. The score for each step was transferred to the spokes of a spider diagram, each divided from 1–10. Once scoring was done, a visual picture of the degree (scope) of participation and empowerment emerged and could be used for comparison with other spider diagrams. To obtain a quantitative measure for participation and empowerment the area inside each spider diagram was calculated.

Laverack (1999) initially used a rating scale to make a participatory assessment of his nine domains called an 'empowerment assessment rating scale (EARS)'. All five statements were written on one sheet. The EARS represented the various levels of community empowerment from the least empowering statement as the first item to the most empowering statement as the last item. A response categorization was attributed to each item. These were given as both fixed alternative expressions (unacceptable, very unsatisfactory, unsatisfactory, satisfactory and most satisfactory), and as weightings of 0, 1, 2, 3, 4. An example of the EAR scale for 'problem assessment' is provided in Table 6.1.

Once the rating scales had been drafted for each domain it was necessary to determine their validity and reliability. Validity refers to how well the scales assess what they are intended to assess. The validity of the proposed EARS, then, refers to whether each scale item is an actual measure of that particular domain. The other issue in regard to the design of the scales is one of internal consistency. This refers to whether the five scale items are sufficiently interrelated and together comprise the concept of that particular domain (Bryman 1992).

Examples of the types of validity that can be used to assess rating scales are *face validity* and *content validity*. Face validity is based on a review by independent people to determine their views on whether the items look

Table 6.1 An example of the EAR scale for 'problem assessment'

0	1	2	3	4
Unacceptable	*Very unsatisfactory*	*Unsatisfactory*	*Satisfactory*	*Most satisfactory*
No problem assessment undertaken	Done by agent. Community lacks skills and awareness to carry out an assessment	Community has skills. Problems and priorities identified by community. Did not involve participation of all sectors of community	Community identified problems, solutions and actions. Assessment used to strengthen community planning	Community continues to identify, and is the owner of, problems, solutions and actions

satisfactory, for example through an informal networking strategy using email. Content validity is a more systematic measure of how appropriate the items seem to a set of identified reviewers who have an understanding of the subject matter. The purpose is for these people to provide insight into the design of the scales based on their own experiences and knowledge (Litwin 1995).

Laverack (1999) found that when the EARS was first applied it was found to influence the behaviour and actions of the participants. The design had led the participants into making the selection of a statement for each domain rather than allowing them to fully reflect on the actual situation in the community. He therefore decided to remove any reference to the rating, including the terminology 'EARS'. The design was further adapted to utilize an approach in which the participants are provided with five statements, each written on a separate sheet of paper. The sheets of paper were not numbered or marked in any way. The absence of any numbering or marking to indicate a rating scale on the sheets meant that the participants were not influenced in the selection. Instead, each statement had to be carefully considered on its own merits by the participants. The participants were able to discard some of the statements and spent time discussing others before reaching a consensus about any particular one.

The visual representation of the evaluation of empowerment

The purpose of visual representation is to provide a means by which to share the analysis and interpretation of the evaluation with all the stakeholders. The information may have to be compared over a specific timeframe and between the different components of a programme. For this purpose, visual representations that are culturally sensitive and easy to reproduce are an appropriate way to interpret and share qualitative information.

Community empowerment is a complex concept which can be viewed and measured as a process that is influenced by nine distinct domains (discussed in Chapter 5). Each domain is measured with five statements that range from the least to the most empowering situation and are rated 1–5. The statements for each domain are also provided in Chapter 5.

The ranking allows each domain to be quantified using a numerical value from 1–5. It is important to remember that this value provides an approximation for a particular domain based on the knowledge and experiences of the participants in relation to the situation in their community at the time of the evaluation. The numerical values can then be visually represented.

The spider-web configuration

The spider-web configuration is specifically designed to be used with the domains approach, as discussed in Chapter 5, for the visual representation of community empowerment. The spider-web configuration is constructed by using readily available computer spreadsheet packages that allow quantitative information to be graphically displayed, usually using the Chart Wizard option. The spider-web configuration is selected from the standard 'radar' type chart and then follows the simple Chart Wizard steps to set the data range, the chart options and the chart location. The visual representation provides a 'snapshot' of the strengths and weaknesses of each domain and of community empowerment as a whole. This information can be used to compare progress within a community and between communities in the same programme. The ratings used to measure community empowerment are relative to changes in the same scale by the same community or between different communities as similarities or differences over a specific timeframe.

Graphing differences over time allows conclusions to be drawn about the effectiveness of building community empowerment in a programme context. The community members and the outside agent can provide a textual analysis to accompany the visual representation to explain why some domains are strong and others are not. The visual and textual analysis can be used to develop strategies to build community empowerment during a specific period, such as between programme reporting cycles (Laverack 2006c).

Figure 6.1 provides a simple visual representation of the baseline measurement of community empowerment in the Bukara village in Kyrgyzstan (SLLP 2004). The spider-web configuration shows that all the domains were weak at the particular time of making the measurement, with the exception of 'resource mobilization'. The community had previous experiences of raising funds through selling locally-made crafts at bazaars and therefore rated this domain higher. In particular, the domain 'programme management' was given a weak rating by the community. This was because the programme was new and a good working relationship between the community and the outside agents had not yet been established.

Subsequent measurements can be carried out and then further plotted onto the same spider-web configuration. Over the lifetime of the programme a visual representation of community empowerment, as it increases or decreases, can be plotted. It is important to support the visual representation with a textual analysis of the circumstances contributing to each rating. This is completed by both the community and the outside agent and will provide more depth to the analysis of the measurement of empowerment.

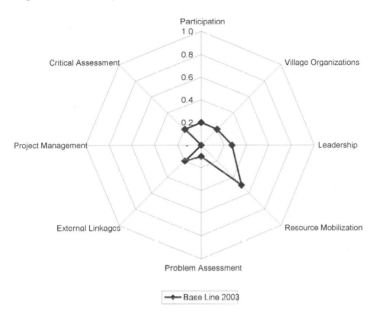

Figure 6.1 Measurement for Bukara village

Figure 6.2 shows the first (baseline) and second measurements of community empowerment in the Tokbai-Talaa village in Kyrgyzstan (SLLP 2004). The two measurements, taken in the same community with the same participants, were made 12 months apart. After the first measurement the community representatives developed a strategic plan to strengthen the domains. In the second measurement there was an improvement in all of the domains with the exception of 'resource mobilization' which remained at the same level. The community representatives decided to develop a strategic plan to strengthen this particular domain over the next six months.

The spider-web in Figure 6.3 provides an example of two measurements, taken in the same community, Ak-Terek in Kyrgyzstan (SLLP 2004), with the

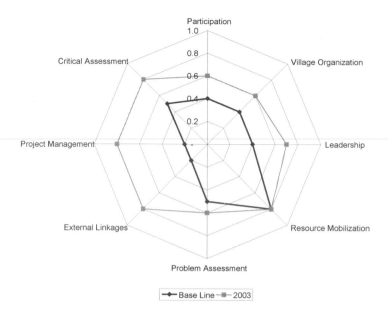

Figure 6.2 Measurements for the Tokbai-Talaa village

same participants, made six months apart. The community's evaluation showed that it had made progress, with the support of the programme, in strengthening all the domains with the exception of 'critical assessment' ('the ability to ask why'). The programme had initially carried out a strengths, weaknesses, opportunities and threats (SWOT) analysis and this included the identification of the immediate needs in the community. However, empowerment requires members of a community to go further than needs assessment and to critically examine the broader (social, political, economic) causes of their powerlessness. This is a crucial stage towards developing appropriate personal and social change strategies and is termed 'critical thinking' and 'critical assessment'. It demonstrates the ability of the community to look outwards and to think contextually rather than continuing to focus on internal and local issues. Strategies such as 'Photovoice' (Wang *et al.* 1998) have been developed to strengthen the critical reflection of a community and could be used as an approach in the Ak-Terek community.

Programmes in which there are more than one community can make a baseline for community empowerment as an average value for each domain of each measurement. Figure 6.4 shows the visual representation in two communities, Aral and Chech Dobo, in the same programme in Kyrgyzstan (SLLP 2004). The measurement of community empowerment has been compared with an average value 'baseline' taken from the other

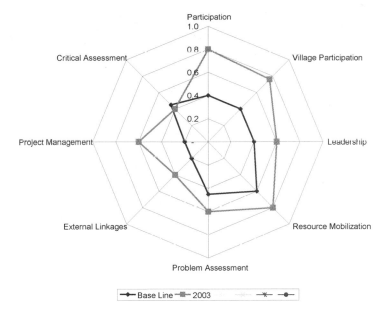

Figure 6.3 Spider-web for Ak-Terek village

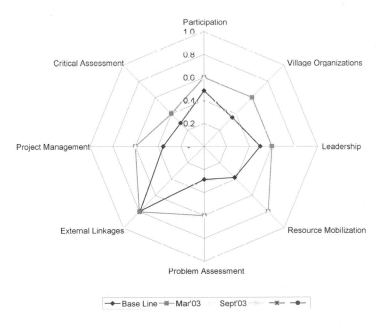

Figure 6.4 Spider-web for Aral and Chech Dobo villages

measurements in the programme to give a comparison across the nine domains. In this way, the progress of any particular community in building empowerment can be assessed against other activities in other communities in the same programme.

The spider-web configuration can also be used to cross-check self-evaluation by the community. If the measurement of each domain is considered to be too high (ratings of 4 and above), the outside agent, in collaboration with the community, can undertake an 'independent' evaluation (Laverack 2006c). This is not totally independent because the co-worker (the outside agent) will have an insight into the community. The spider-web in Figure 6.5 shows an example of an evaluation by two women's groups in Nepal. The ratings for all the domains were high in both communities and a third 'independent' evaluation was carried out by the health worker to cross-check the findings. It confirmed that the high ratings of each domain made by the women's groups were correct (Gibbon *et al.* 2002).

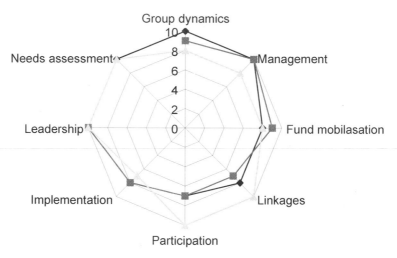

Figure 6.5 Cross-checking the measurement of community empowerment

Adapting the spider-web configuration

Kirsten Havemann (2006), a researcher and practitioner, undertook a pilot study to develop and test methods for data collection and analysis of participation and empowerment. Her study used an adaptation of the domains approach and the spider-web configuration. The aim of the study, which was part of an ongoing countrywide community-based programme in Kenya, was to establish village-based institutions that could act as vehicles for improving livelihoods through empowerment. The sampling frame for the pilot study included all the residents of Mazumalume and Simkumbe sublocations of Kwale District with a total sampling frame of 19,800 people in 2064 households. The piloting of the tools was done in Mwangane village, Mwatate sublocation, Mwatate location of Samburu division in Kwale district which had a population of 320.

The data collection started with the drawing of village resource and social maps by the research team and a group of 12 villagers. These maps were compared and validated with maps previously drawn by the villagers during the initiation of the project. Key informants, such as the traditional birth attendant, the community health worker and the traditional healer, were identified using the social map and then interviewed. The research team did a transect walk through the village in order to verify the newly-drawn maps, but also to get to know the villagers and interview the identified key informants. For ease of planning, a checklist of places to visit and people to be interviewed was prepared prior to the transect walk.

The sub-chief and the village chairman then called for a *Baraza* or community meeting. The participants were divided into three groups: a mixed gender group, a female group and a group of children. It was not possible to get a male group due to the poor attendance rate of men. Each group was asked to answer the following seven questions:

1 In which step, if any, did the methods you learned help you to participate in health development?
2 Which step, if any, has mostly influenced your behaviour/attitude towards better health?
3 Which step, if any, has mostly contributed to you sharing your health knowledge and skills in the community?
4 Which step, if any, has been the most important for improving your access to resources contributing to better health?
5 Which step, if any, has contributed most to institutional change (mainly with reference to the Ministry of Health) for better health?
6 Which step, if any, has contributed most to your personal change for better health?
7 Which step, if any, has enabled you (the community) to control resources for better health outcomes?

Sixty stones were collected four times and the villagers were asked to give a score out of ten for each of the seven questions. This was according to the felt importance each step had in contributing to their participation and/or empowerment in the health development activities. For the purpose of visualization and calculation of an overall effectiveness score of participation and empowerment, the score for each step was transferred to the spokes of a spider diagram (each divided into ten) by the research facilitation team. Two of the diagrams are shown in Figures 6.6 (empowerment) and 6.7 (participation).

Once the scoring was done, a visual picture of the degree of participation and empowerment emerged and could be used for comparison with other spider diagrams. To obtain a quantitative measure for participation and empowerment the area inside each spider diagram was calculated. This area was already divided into eight triangles by the nature of the spider. The following formula for calculating the sum of the areas of these eight triangles was developed and used:

$$\text{Area } 1 = \tfrac{\sqrt{2}}{4}\,[X_1 \cdot X_2 + X_2 \cdot X_3 + X_3 \cdot X_4 + X_4 \cdot X_5 + X_5 \cdot X_6 + X_6 \cdot X_7 + X_7 \cdot X_8 + X_8 \cdot X_1]$$

Area 1 measures the scope of participation and is the total sum area inside the spider diagram resulting from adding the sum of the eight triangles. 'X' is the scored value from one of the steps in the health development process transferred to a spoke on the spider diagram. It should be noted that the focus on numbers and equations runs a real risk of deflecting attention away from the process of empowerment. The spider diagram is a simple means of visual representation and interpretation. It is not to be depended upon as a means of quantifying or measuring specific outcomes for each domain.

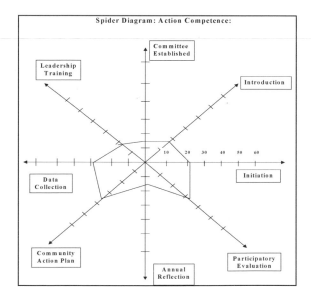

Figure 6.6   Spider diagram for empowerment

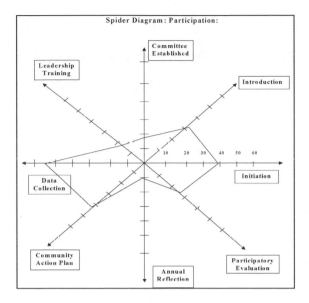

Figure 6.7 Spider diagram for participation

Chapter 7 discusses how the 'domains approach' has been used to build community empowerment to address issue-based approaches in health promotion programming and uses case study examples from two different contexts.

7 Empowerment in action: an issues-based approach

This chapter discusses two case study examples of how to build community empowerment by using the nine domains discussed in Chapter 5 within an issues-based approach to health promotion programming. The two case studies are 'Improving health outcomes and community capacity in Canada' and 'Improving housing standards in an inner city area in England'.

In health promotion theory, communities are often positioned as requiring the assistance of an outside agent to help them to identify and address their needs. In practice, communities often already know what they want, based on a shared understanding of their issues and problems. However, communities sometimes do not know how to resolve their problems or issues. To achieve this involves a process of capacity-building that may, or may not, lead the community to become empowered. The term 'problem assessment' is often used in health promotion because communities identify specific problems about which they are concerned, in contrast to the outside agents who usually think in terms of community 'needs'. Communities prefer the terms 'problems' or 'issues' because they can see the possibility of resolving them. Whatever term is used, an assessment is most empowering when the identification of, and the solutions to, a resolution are carried out by the community.

The first case study discusses attempts to improve health outcomes at the same time as building community capacity. In an innovative way, a community-based issue, physical activity, was used as an entry point to develop a broader agenda on health.

Case study 1: improving health outcomes and community capacity in Canada

The Saskatoon 'In Motion Programme'

Bell-Woodard et al. (2005), four health promotion researchers in Canada, present the findings of a study that included key stakeholder groups responsible for a physical activity programme, the 'Saskatoon In Motion Programme' (called here 'SIMP'). The purpose was to provide an overall assessment of the community impact of such an initiative in terms of health outcomes and community capacity-building.

In 1999, four agencies in a mid-sized Canadian city, Saskatoon (the Regional Health Authority; the City of Saskatoon, a major provider of recreational programmes and facilities in the community; the University of Saskatchewan, specifically the College of Kinesiology; and ParticipACTION, a national physical activity promotion organization) formed a partnership to develop and implement the community-wide active living initiative (SIMP). The mandate of this initiative was to unite the strengths of public, private, academic and industry efforts into a collaborative alliance to inspire the residents of Saskatoon to lead physically active lives that would enhance their health and quality of life. The capacity-building element examined community-wide changes and outcomes not directly linked to physical exercise, but rather as a result of the implementation of the SIMP. The nine domains (Laverack 1999 and Chapter 5) were used as indicators for the measurement of community capacity. These domains had been field-tested in a number of different countries with health promotion and development projects (Gibbon et al. 2002).

The first stage was a workshop hosted by the outside agent (the researchers) to acquaint the partners with community capacity and its assessment. A review of the developmental history of the initiative was presented to ensure partners had a shared and agreed upon understanding of their own recent past. This was followed by descriptions of capacity-building concepts and consensus agreement by the partners on definitions for the nine capacity domains. Five descriptive indicators on a continuum for each domain were created specifically for the SIMP (see Box 7.1 for an example). The indicators ranged from minimal/absent (1) to fully realized/optimal (5) and this numerical scaling was used to provide a comparison between domains over time. Following the workshop, this Likert-like measurement tool was completed by each partner independently and returned to the researcher. Aggregate results of the partners' assessments, including means, range of scores and comments were collated. The comments generated were an integral part of the methodology as they represented information offered by the partners in support of their assessments. Following this baseline assessment, over the next year the outside agent continued to observe and interact with the co-ordinating committee as well as the various action committees of the SIMP, collecting reflective notes on meetings and events.

Another workshop with the partners was hosted a year later at which time a second rating of community capacity was completed. The previous year's means and results were available to the partners. There were some changes to the methodology used at this workshop in an effort to streamline, simplify and enrich the process. These included having the partners complete the assessment at the workshop (to avoid the delay of returning assessments) and eliminating the organizational assessment of the SIMP (since participants were unable to rate both community capacity and the initiative). An opportunity was given to the partners to engage in a more extensive discussion of the domains and their effects on programme sustainability, as based on the previous year's assessment, and much of the 'richness' of the data emerged through this technique.

Box 7.1 An example of a domain definition and indicators

Problem assessment is the ability of a community to assess needs and assets using all available evidence, based on its values, to determine actions to solve a problem.

Indicators for problem assessment

1 The community is unaware that a problem exists.
2 The community is aware that the problem of physical inactivity exists, but lacks the skills and confidence to do something.
3 The community is aware of the problem, and they have some skills and support to undertake action.
4 The community is beginning to identify solutions and take some action.
5 The community considers itself the 'owner' of the problem of physical inactivity, and is continuously revising the issue, coming up with solutions and taking action (Bell-Woodard *et al.* 2005).

Subsequent to the first assessment a series of interviews (n = 10) with external community agencies and individuals who had had some contact with the SIMP was completed as a validity check on the partners' assessment. Agencies included school consultants and teachers, private fitness providers, action committee members, professionals interested in physical activity (physiotherapists, nurses), public health staff, community fundraisers and members of inner-city community action groups. They were asked about overall community changes that were a result of the SIMP and about specific changes in each of the domains. In addition, they commented on the influence physical activity had on the initiative's success, the challenges they saw, and provided their perspectives on the sustainability of the SIMP. Data gathered from the partners, the external agency respondents and participant observations by the primary researcher were content analysed, subjected to face validity checks with other researchers involved with other studies pertaining to the SIMP and, with implications and recommendations, provided to the partners.

The impact of the SIMP

What impact did this physical activity health promotion programme have on community capacity? Table 7.1 summarizes the numerical results of the capacity assessments completed by the partners for the Saskatoon community in Years 1 and 2.

Table 7.1 Capacity assessment of the community of Saskatoon

Domain	Year 1 Assessment (mean) N = 9	Year 1 Range	Year 2 Assessment (mean) N = 9	Year 2 Range
Stakeholder participation	3.03	2.0–5.0	4.4	3.8–5.0
Local leadership	3.4	1.8–4.5	4.2	2.0–4.5
Organizational structures	3.7	2.5–5.0	4.1	3.8–4.9
Problem assessment	3.2	2.3–4.3	3.8	3.0–4.2
Resource mobilization	3.1	2.0–4.5	3.9	2.8–4.9
'Asking why'	3.2	2.0–4.5	3.7	3.0–4.0
Links with others	Not rated #		3.7*	2.0–4.6
Role of outside agents	3.4	2.0–5.0	3.8	3.0–4.3
Programme management	2.7	1.8–5.0	3.1	2.0–4.0

* One respondent reordered the continuum of indicators in this domain. # Partners ran out of time to rate this domain.

Source: Bell-Woodard *et al.* (2005)

The combined data sources from this study indicate that the SIMP has drawn on a shared vision, and benefited from experienced and influential leadership. The programme identified a number of local leaders including:

- Catholic bishop's leadership in initiatives focusing on older adults;
- school division leadership, including consultants, board policies and administration support in children and youth initiatives;
- corporate leadership;
- neighbourhood leadership in youth ands adult groups;
- older adults action committee identifies leadership recruitment as a need and obtains resources to train leaders.

The initiative successfully gathered evidence to contribute to problem assessment. Stakeholders (partners) came on board and maintained a commitment to the initiative for over five years and new stakeholders in the community were engaged. Resources have been mobilized and communication with the community has been strong. Leadership is continuing to be developed. The elements of a capacity-building model that are perhaps less well developed include sustainable organizational structures for growth, the influence of the initiative on policies, and critical analysis skills for the further development of the programme.

The SIMP also demonstrated a positive impact on physical activity as several respondents noted:

> everybody is trapped in their body ... so everyone is connected personally. Other issues such as child prostitution are philosophical and need policy responses that can only be achieved through education. But with physical activity, people can change it themselves.

> this is a fun thing and the majority of the population can see and apply what the programme means personally.
>
> (Bell-Woodard *et al*. 2005: 10)

There is evidence that the success of this partnership around physical activity has led to spin-offs in other community processes. For example, the planning for a new neighbourhood and the establishment of a primary health care site have both included consideration of physical activity needs. The SIMP demonstrated that a physical activity health promotion programme can also function to build community capacity (Bell-Woodard *et al*. 2005: 13).

The study concluded by saying that notwithstanding the limitations of a relatively new methodology, the methods and measurements of community capacity assessment used offer a defensible and useful approach to health promotion evaluation. Moreover, and perhaps more importantly, the general approach of continuous accompaniment, stakeholder involvement in the development of measurement tools, regular feedback to the partners' group and theoretical grounding created participatory research that was also useful to the initiative in guiding its ongoing development.

The second case study is based on the experiences of the author in terms of how an issues-based approach (social housing in a deprived inner-city area of England) can be addressed through each of the nine empowerment domains.

Case study 2: improving housing standards in an inner-city area in England

A residents' association of older people situated in a deprived housing estate in Leeds, West Yorkshire, England, was fed up with their poor living conditions. The housing in the area was a mixture of low- and high-rise accommodation, some privately owned and some rented. The urban area faced problems of high unemployment and antisocial behaviour such as vandalism and street crime, and had a dilapidated infrastructure with poor street lighting and faulty lifts in some of the high-rise buildings.

Dominant images of older people in a particular period of time and place are held by society. Today's dominant image of ageing is of frailty, helplessness and dependency, and the professional 'problem' of ageing is an issue of dependency and care. In reality, many older people do not suffer severe disability and are not dependent on others. Discrimination against older people therefore rests on a pathology model which focuses on social isolation, poverty, illness, unemployment and bereavement. These negative perceptions can also direct government policy on the distribution of resources for the aged. Older persons can internalize these perceptions and this contributes to a lower self-esteem and feelings of helplessness (Onyx and Benton 1995).

The health promotion practitioners in this case study were aware of the direct effects of poverty and deprived housing on the sense of hopelessness, isolation and self-blame of older people living in such conditions. The practitioners believed that older persons are the best advocates for their own empowerment and that this can begin with the actions of individuals who suffer the inequalities of poor housing. To change their situation they are compelled to gain access to power by participating in interest groups – for example, the residents' association – that share their concerns. They may have to build their power from within first to have the confidence to participate in a group setting in such a way as to make their opinions count. Older people can increase their level of participation through the gradual development of their social skills, by belonging to a network of self-help and interest groups, by seeking advice, through education and training, and by becoming more aware of their rights and connecting with others with similar political concerns.

Representatives of the residents' association met one afternoon in a room provided at the local health centre to discuss how they could address their problems. They decided to invite the local health promotion practitioner to help them to make a strategic plan to address the main issue: improving living and housing standards. Epidemiological studies have shown an association between poor housing and health (Thomson *et al.* 2001) but the small size of sample populations and a lack of control for confounders limit the generalization of these findings. However, the basic human need for proper housing and the relationship between poor living conditions and poor health are obvious to many practitioners working in this type of environment. The health promotion practitioner, at the request of the residents' association, therefore decided to go ahead and to support their proposal to help empower older people to improve their housing standards.

Individuals have a better chance of success in addressing the broader inequalities in their lives if they can act collectively. It is through collective action that people can increase their access to resources, influence decisions and build support through wider participation. It is governments that create the policies that are largely responsible for the distribution of resources for older people. By increasing their membership and resource base, the residents' association felt it would be better able to have an influence on government policy.

The association decided to firstly improve the level of community participation on the issue of deprived housing. This was to provide an entry point into the community to develop a broader agenda on health and housing. The practitioner, who attended the first meeting, recommended that they carefully consider each of the nine domains to help them to make a plan to build participation, and the other areas of influence, for future development. This plan would then be submitted for government funding as part of a health promotion programme. The representatives of the association also identified a number of questions that could be asked to help the community to take more control of the proposed health promotion programme. The development of a plan was an ongoing process of discussion and critical thinking by the community representatives and this was facilitated at each meeting by the practitioner.

Applying the empowerment domains to the community issue

Improves participation. Urging people to simply attend classroom-style education sessions is less likely to attract participation than organizing events based around community members' interests. The programme should initially organize people around what they have identified as being important to them in the design phase, implemented as activities that they like to do – for example, social and exercise groups for older people. The practitioner facilitated a discussion of concerns that the people, who were mostly women, would like to continue meeting about, such as the lack of locally available fitness facilities. The issue of fitness and body image generated a lot of discussion and was suggested as a good theme. It involved action, not just discussion, and would promote participation.

The residents' association asked the following questions in regard to participation during its meetings:

- Are individuals actively involved in community groups?
- How are community groups and organizations actively involved in the programme?
- Are all community members and groups of the targeted population represented in the community participation – for example, attending meetings?
- Has the practitioner helped the community to identify all potential barriers to participation?
- How is the programme addressing the barriers to participation?
- How is the practitioner helping to maintain participation?

Develops local leadership. Developing local leaders means working with and building on existing strengths and community capacities. If a leader is not available the programme may support local volunteers with good networks, organizing and building leadership qualities. The new leaders must at least have the support of other local leaders and of the members of the community, for example through an elective process. The programme used local volunteers with good organizing and planning skills in neighbourhood activities such as bingo and other social events. In most communities, leaders are historically and culturally determined and programmes which ignore this have little chance of success.

The residents' association asked the following questions in regard to leadership during its meetings:

- How has the practitioner helped the local leaders to identify their needs?
- How is the practitioner supporting leadership in community-based organizations?
- Do leaders have clearly defined roles within the implementation of the programme?
- Are leaders accountable within the programme?

Builds empowering organizational structures. The practitioner realized that the locality lacked strong community structures and used the fitness group and neighbourhood activities to lay the framework for a new organization. It may not always be necessary to create a new organization, but if there are no organizations sufficiently representative of community members, a new one may have to be developed. The new organization need not be restricted to one mandate but may wish to begin with a single issue that is relevant to the participants. Any existing organizations should be strengthened by the new one and not compete against it.

The residents' association asked the following questions in regard to organizational structures during its meetings:

- How has the practitioner helped the community-based organizations to identify their needs?
- How is the programme utilizing existing community organizations?
- How is the practitioner helping to establish the structure of the organization (formal membership, goals, budget, reporting etc.)?
- How is the practitioner helping to promote equity and participation in the organizations?
- How is the practitioner helping to develop the skills of the members of community organizations?
- Have the organizations got clearly defined roles and responsibilities within the programme?

Increases problem assessment capacities. The association already knew a great deal about local issues. The practitioner helped to engage community members in a broader form of problem assessment, one that incorporated their immediate issues, such as safe road crossing areas and the broader problems in their neighbourhood, such as security. This information became the basis of planning new activities, both short-term (to keep participation active) and long-term (to work on underlying causes such as the lack of youth employment). The outside agent can help to engage community members in a broader form of problem assessment, one that incorporates both capacities and problems in the neighbourhood (e.g. what makes people in this area healthy, what makes them ill?). Specifically designed tools for mapping, both short-term and long-term are available elsewhere (see Laverack 2005: 48).

The association asked the following questions in regard to problem assessment during its meetings:

- How has the practitioner assisted the community to identify its own problems and concerns?
- How is the practitioner helping the community to address these problems and concerns?
- How have these problems and concerns been built into the design of the programme?
- How will these problems and concerns be monitored and evaluated?

Enhances the ability to 'ask why'. Rather than using an education approach the practitioner decided to help the residents by working with them to analyse why some people had poorer health and others did not, why some people had unhealthy living conditions and others did not, and what local, state and national actions might remedy their particular circumstances. This helped them to increase their level of understanding and was developed further by using tools to promote critical reflection (Wang and Pies 2004) in small groups.

The association asked the following questions in regard to 'asking why' during its meetings:

- How is the practitioner helping people to come together in groups to identify the underlying causes of their powerlessness and poverty?
- What 'tools' and approaches is the practitioner using to help raise the consciousness of people about the underlying causes of their powerlessness and poverty?
- How is the practitioner helping people to identify solutions to the underlying causes of their powerlessness and poverty?
- How is the practitioner helping people to gain experience of implementing the solutions to the underlying causes of their powerlessness?

Improves resource mobilization. The programme came with some resources that were committed to conventional community development outcomes such as increasing participation. The practitioner used some of her own time and funding to support the broader-based organizing that she had helped initiate in the community. More importantly, the residents' association and the practitioner worked together to attract resources for outcomes of a community development programme in a deprived housing area. It is important that the members prioritize raising resources as this will develop their sense of ownership and commitment and will give programme activities a better chance of sustainability. The community can start to raise internal resources on a small scale through fundraising (e.g. a sponsored walk) and raise external resources through seeking outside funding (e.g. from government grants for healthy urbanization). Some issues may fall outside what funders consider to be legitimate activities for health promotion and disease prevention (e.g. the provision of refreshments and travel costs for representatives to support a social event).

The association asked the following questions in regard to resource mobilization during its meetings:

- How is the practitioner helping the community to identify the resources that it needs within the programme?
- How is the practitioner helping the community to identify its resource base?
- How is the practitioner helping the community to mobilize internal resources?
- How is the practitioner helping the community to mobilize external resources?
- How is the practitioner helping with the equitable distribution of the resources within the programme?

- How is the use of these resources accountable within the programme?

Strengthens links to other organizations and people. The practitioner was interested in linking the residents' association with others undertaking similarly broad-based, local organizing. This included brokering ties with local politicians and policy-makers (especially concerning health-housing risk conditions) and was supported by advocacy on these issues through the practitioner's own agency and professional statements. The practitioner can also provide contact addresses, emails and website links that could develop into a more proactive strategy to link to other communities. Visits to meet and exchange experiences are important to gain additional information, or the practitioner can arrange for a guest speaker to come to the community to discuss their successes and failures in similar programmes. Communities sometimes feel that they are working in isolation and it is good for the practitioner to help the members to understand how the difficulties that they face may have been overcome by others.

The association asked the following questions in regard to links to others during its meetings:

- How is the practitioner helping the residents' association to establish a network with other communities, organizations and people?
- What information has the practitioner provided to help establish links with other communities, organizations and people (websites, telephone numbers etc.)?
- Has the practitioner organized any experience exchange activities with other communities, organizations and people?
- How has the practitioner helped to establish formal links with other communities, organizations and people (e.g. by defining roles and responsibilities)?
- What outcomes have been achieved through establishing links with other communities, organizations and people?
- How is the networking with others built into the design of the programme?
- How are the links with other communities, organizations and people being monitored and evaluated by the programme?

Creates an equitable relationship with outside agents and increases control over programme management. The primary outside agent in this programme, the practitioner, maintained critical self-reflection on their own role: Were they imposing? Facilitating? Empowering? This ongoing self-assessment was supported by their agency manager, and evaluated periodically through discussion with community members. Over time, and as additional resources were obtained, the residents' association took more direct control over their activities. Here, control is generalized to the broader range of organizing efforts such as administration, finance and management. What is important is the way in which support is provided by the outside agent. The support should be at the request of the residents' association and should aim to build community capacities and be delivered as a partnership with community members.

The association asked the following questions in regard to an equitable relationship with the practitioner during its meetings:

- How is the residents' association actively involved in the design of the programme?
- How are the outside agency and practitioner devolving responsibility to the residents' association for programme implementation, management and evaluation?
- Has the practitioner established clear roles and responsibilities for the residents' association within the programme?
- How will the practitioner ensure that decision-making mechanisms between the association and the programme management are equitable?
- How are the outside agency and practitioner ensuring that the association has the necessary skills to manage the programme?
- How are the outside agency and practitioner ensuring that the association has the necessary resources to support their inputs in the programme?

The short-term success of the programme would be evaluated by improvements in the initial community activities, such as exercise activities. The medium-term success would be evaluated by improvements in goals set by the residents' association, such as establishing a more secure environment. The long-term success would be an increase in the residents' association's activities to enhance its ability to question the underlying reasons for the issues it wants to address such as poor housing and its contribution toward changes in housing policy and legislation (Laverack 2006a). This latter success is achieved through building the capacity of the association in each of the nine domains, for example, increasing participation, developing the organization and developing social support. The legitimate actions of the association can be used to influence government decisions, for example, by registering a complaint to a local authority, by placing their name on a petition in protest against the housing conditions in which they live and by writing a letter to their Member of Parliament or a local newspaper. The association could also take more direct actions such as legal action against landlords and demonstrating and protesting against those it feels are the cause of the poor housing. These activities can be facilitated by an outside agent such as the health promotion practitioner. The purpose is to build the capacity of the older people to assist them to have a greater sense of control in their lives.

Chapter 8 provides two case studies of how the empowerment domains can be used to address community-based approaches in health promotion programmes: improving health in a rural community in Northern Australia and improving livelihoods in rural communities in Kyrgyzstan.

8 Empowerment in action: a community-based approach

This chapter discusses two case study examples that allow practitioners to better understand how to build community empowerment by using the nine empowerment domains within a community-based approach in health promotion programmes. The two case studies are 'Improving health and hygiene in a remote community in Northern Australia' and 'Improving livelihoods in rural communities in Kyrgyzstan'.

Chapter 7 discussed how to build community empowerment within an issues-based approach. The two approaches, issues-based and community-based, are closely linked in empowerment because it is the 'community' that identifies the issues to be addressed. However, in health promotion programming there is often a distinction made in the focus between either a specific issue and/or a defined community. In an issues-based approach it is the 'issue', for example, physical exercise, that is the focus for the programme design. In a community-based approach it is the 'community' (defined in Chapter 2) which provides the focus for the programme design.

The notion of health promotion operating in a context beyond individually-defined issues or problems was in part responsible for the emergence of a settings-based approach in the 1990s. This was also the result of a theoretical shift in emphasis from individual health issues and topic-based 'risk factors' to the nature of 'the system' and 'the organization' as relatively complex phenomena. Consequently, a range of settings-based movements were developed – for example, healthy cities, healthy islands, workplaces, schools, health care and clinic settings and, as discussed in this chapter, communities (Whitelaw *et al.* 2001).

Case study 1: improving health and hygiene in a remote community in Northern Australia

Aboriginal communities in Australia are often a collection of families, language groups or clans who can be in competition over limited resources and who may traditionally have been geographically isolated. Once living a nomadic and rural lifestyle, Aboriginal people now mostly live in urban areas where they form a minority group. However, many Aboriginal people still live in rural communities. The term 'community' was applied to the formation of the settlements or 'Aboriginal reserves' by bureaucratic intellectuals and those in authority because it provided a convenient label for the assimilation of a heterogeneous group of people (Scrimgeour 1997). Aboriginal people experience a health status well below the Australian average – for example, for indicators of child survival rates, birth weight and the growth and nutrition of babies. This has been related to their poor psychological health resulting from cultural disintegration, dispossession of their lands, unemployment and poverty (O'Connor and Parker 1995), and to poor sanitary conditions associated with poor housing design and living conditions (Laverack 2000).

This case study describes how a remote Aboriginal community was used as the focus for a programme to strengthen community empowerment (Laverack 2000). To protect the privacy of the members of the community the names of individuals and the identity of the location have not been used.

The health promotion context

The community is situated in a rural location approximately eight hours drive east of Darwin in the Northern Territory of Australia. It has an estimated population of 970 residents, predominately Aboriginal. Following a discussion with the community council and elders the Environmental Health Services undertook a programme to promote health in regard to hygiene standards in tenanted houses. Housing was differentiated into three types of 'domestic unit' (see Lots 1, 2 and 3 below). A 'domestic unit' or household can be described as 'a wide range of people' including visiting relatives, individuals, young men and 'family units'. A 'family unit' is described as two adults and a number of children and/or a relative (Willis 1987).

Housing type Lot 1

Lot 1 is a small domestic unit (not more than five people), consisting of one family unit and relatives in which the head of the household has clear authority and cleaning is shared by the occupants. As a consequence the house was clean, functional, well maintained and its occupants took pride in its appearance. Lot 1 has four bedrooms, a central communal living area, bathroom, toilet and laundry tub and a covered veranda at the front and rear of the house. Lot 1 was occupied by five people who formed one family unit: the father, mother, two children and a male relative. The fixtures and fittings of the house were all functional although the occupants did not own a washing machine or a refrigerator. To wash clothes the occupants used the public laundromat facility that is within 250 metres of the house. In terms of repair Lot 1 was not the best house in the community but had a high standard of repair.

Lot 1 was considered by its occupants to be a 'strong house', one which had clear lines of authority and responsibility. These were delegated by the father, the head of the household, who took responsibility for the division of labour for cleaning and maintaining the house. The house was not over-crowded and communal areas such as the kitchen and bathroom were shared and kept very clean. Cleaning was carried out by the adult occupants of the house including the male relative, who was responsible for keeping his own bedroom clean.

Housing type Lot 2

Lot 2 is a domestic unit (not more than ten people) consisting of two or more family units in which cleaning responsibility is shared among the occupants or is delegated to a few people. Lot 2 is a similarly designed four-bedroom house to Lot 1. It has a central communal living area, bathroom, toilet and laundry tub and a covered veranda at the front and rear of the house. Lot 2 is occupied by nine people who form one domestic unit and consists of two family units; mother, father and children and other relatives. The household facilities were functional, although the occupants did not own a washing machine but did have a refrigerator. The house was especially dirty in the communal kitchen, bathroom and toilet areas.

The head of the household and his wife both felt that cleaning should be a shared responsibility of everyone occupying the house. However, guests or relatives of the domestic unit who were living in the house for a temporary but indefinite period were not asked to contribute toward cleaning.

Aboriginal households encompass a wide range of people, spread over a large geographical area, and this can result in many visitors to the domestic unit from, for example, other communities and out-stations. In practice many occupants in medium domestic units do not have an obligation to actively help with the responsibility of cleaning. Instead these chores are the responsibility of a few female occupants of the family unit(s), along with the many other onerous duties they have to perform.

With an occupancy level bordering on overcrowding, the women responsible for cleaning in Lot 2 found it increasingly difficult to maintain cleanliness. Periodic spring-cleaning of the house, sometimes shared by other occupants, did help to maintain cleanliness. However, unsanitary conditions were a continual risk to health and could quickly arise when cleaning had to be given a lower priority in the event of circumstances such as caring for a sick person or travelling to attend a ceremony.

Housing type Lot 3

Lot 3 is a large domestic unit (more than 10 and up to 25 people) consisting of many 'family units', relatives and groups in which responsibility for cleaning was not equally shared but was periodically performed by a few people and authority was ill-defined. Lot 3 is a similarly designed four-bedroom house to

Lots 1 and 2 and has a central communal living area, bathroom, toilet and laundry tub at the rear and a covered veranda at the front and rear of the house. Lot 3 is occupied by 25 people who form one domestic unit that is made up of many different individuals, family units and groups living in a communal setting.

Lot 3 had a low standard of cleanliness throughout the house and in particular the communal areas such as the bathroom, kitchen and toilet were unsanitary. Responsibility for cleaning, both inside and outside the house, was performed by a few women belonging to family units occupying the house. Guests did not participate in cleaning. The workload of cleaning a house occupied by 25 people, in addition to other duties such as cooking, washing and child care, was enormous. The occupants of Lot 3 recognized that the sheer number of people was sufficient to create unhealthy conditions. The division of labour for cleaning communal areas of the house such as the kitchen, toilet and bathroom was not clearly defined, a situation that was further complicated by the head of the household whose authority was shared with the other senior member of the domestic unit.

In Lot 3 the communal areas of the house gradually became untidy and unclean as more people utilized these facilities but did not contribute to their cleanliness. When conditions became unsanitary and intolerable the occupants organized the cleaning of the communal areas, often with the help of others, to provide a better living environment. However, the standard of cleanliness in the house generally remained low and was a risk to health through poor domestic hygiene. The underlying cause of this uncleanliness was the high occupancy level of the house.

The community members concluded that it was high occupancy levels and overcrowded communal living conditions that were the most influential factors on housing repair and standards of hygiene. For example, houses of a similar size and design (Lots 1, 2 and 3) were often shown to be clean and well maintained when they had a low occupancy level but were unsanitary when overcrowded. Unsanitary conditions were most common in those houses that exceeded the prescribed overcrowding standard.

High occupancy levels and overcrowded communal living conditions also have important implications for the lines of authority in regard to cleaning responsibility and domestic hygiene. The head of the household, whose authority may be traditionally used to delegate responsibilities for activities such as cleaning, was clear and well defined in small domestic units. However, within the context of overcrowded conditions the authority of the head of the household often became ill-defined and it was unclear to the occupants who had the responsibility to delegate cleaning the communal areas in the house. In overcrowded circumstances, policies to improve housing repairs alone are insufficient to have an impact on health. It is necessary for at least the following three factors to be consecutively addressed:

the state of housing repair, including the provision of facilities; the occupancy levels and communal living arrangements; and the standard of domestic and food hygiene. These factors can be supported by strategies which directly involve the education of householders to ensure access to cleaning materials and to take into account the implications of communal living, responsibility and authority. More importantly, the community needed to take more control over the factors which were influencing their lives, including housing conditions and cleanliness (Laverack 2000).

A community-based approach to promote health and hygiene

To promote the health and empowerment of the community the principles of the *Ottawa Charter for Health Promotion* (WHO 1986) and the nine domains discussed in Chapter 5 were applied (Laverack 2000). Community empowerment is embraced as a key strategy in the *Charter*, which identifies five action areas for achieving better health: building healthy public policy; creating supportive environments; strengthening community action; developing personal skills; and reorienting health services. The *Charter* also refers to enabling people to increase control over, and to improve, their health, as an important role for practitioners. Together, the community and the outside agency should develop a programme to improve domestic and food hygiene in households as follows.

Action area: strengthening community empowerment
The *Ottawa Charter* describes an empowered community as one in which individuals and organizations apply their skills and resources in collective efforts to address health priorities and meet their respective health needs. In practice this means the community increasing control over, and improving the health of, its members through a process of capacity-building using the domains approach.

Participation. All the representatives from the different clans in the community participated in group discussions during the preparation of the programme. Every year a survey of the state of repair of tenanted houses is carried out in many rural communities in the Northern Territory. The survey provides a crude rating of each house in terms of its 'functionality' and identifies the necessary repairs and improvements to maintain the housing stock. In some communities a standardized questionnaire has been used to record the state of repair of each house and the number of occupants. The findings of the survey were shared with the community members who were encouraged to take an active interest in the programme. Regular meetings were held in the community centre to discuss the programme, facilitated by a practitioner, such as an environmental health officer or Aboriginal health promotion officer.

Leadership. At the beginning of the programme the leadership was guided by the practitioners who held regular consultations with community representatives. The Council of Elders and other local leaders are involved in the planning and administration of the programme and receive training and instruction in management skills to build their capacity. The leaders increasingly make decisions concerning the programme with the purpose of devolving responsibility to the community.

Organizational structures. It is important that an existing organization has the overall responsibility to implement the programme. In this case it was the Community Management Board. Other organizational groups within the community were also involved in the discussion of key issues – for example, the local store would need to be consulted to ensure that sufficient cleaning materials were available at an affordable price. To enable people to increase control of, and improve, health through the management and supervision of the programme it was necessary to develop an understanding of the key issues (see 'Developing personal skills' on p. 00).

Problem assessment. The leaders were encouraged to map and prioritize the immediate 'problems' involved in promoting domestic hygiene. These included a lack of participation, money and low skill level in managing a programme of this size. These issues then became the basis for the planning of strategies for decision-making activities and for the identification of the resources necessary to support these new roles.

Asking why. The participants began to identify the underlying causes of their powerlessness and poor health via a facilitated process of small-group meetings. In such cases, the practitioner can stimulate the participants' sense of critical awareness by using techniques such as Photovoice (see Chapter 3). The leaders soon realized that the unsanitary conditions in many households were caused by social and cultural constraints such as the breakdown of authority of the head of the household. The Council of Elders recognized that it was essential to set in place systems for cleaning in each household, depending on the nature of occupancy (Lots 1, 2 or 3). The Elders prepared a schedule of materials required for routine domestic hygiene to help guide each household.

Resource mobilization. The community had access to only limited resources but still had to raise finances to provide cleaning materials such as detergents and soap. Such things can of course be made available at a local store at subsidised prices or a special pack of materials can be delivered to each household free of charge. However, community members are less likely to value materials which have been provided as government 'handouts' and even goods that are available at discounted prices tend to be unpopular because people think they are of an inferior quality. A community can start to raise additional internal resources on a small scale through fundraising and external resources through seeking government funding, assisted by the practitioner. This community was able to access funds from the Regional Health Service for the provision of plastic baby baths for families with children less than 2 years. Some households had been using the kitchen sink to bathe small children which had resulted in accidents.

Links to others. A community can use strategies to develop links with other communities and arrange for visits to exchange experiences. The Council of Elders proposed a working agreement with the local store, which is privately owned, to ensure that certain cleaning materials such as soap and detergents will be available at an affordable price. However, the owner was not in favour of the proposal because previous experience had demonstrated that community members refused to buy discounted goods because they believed them to be inferior.

Outside agents. Practitioners can play an important role in helping the community to raise resources, develop skills and capacities, gain access to policy-makers and support the programme through their own 'expert' and legitimate power – for example, by raising the concerns of the community with government officials.

Programme management. The purpose of programme management is to increasingly give control to the Council of Elders. This includes management, decision-making, administration, fundraising and liaison with government officials. The role of the practitioner should diminish to provide assistance and resource support at the request of the board. The support of the practitioner is especially important at the beginning of a programme when the confidence and skill level of the community members may be low and capacity-building has to be developed.

Action area: building healthy public policy

Decision-makers in the community had the opportunity to support the equality of access to hygiene facilities. The community had public access to ten commercial washing machines and four dryers 24-hours a day. The success of this facility was built upon by the Council of Elders to address the following:

- The recontamination of clothing due to the practice of drying it on the ground can negate the prior removal of harmful bacteria. The existing facility should be extended to include adequate clothes-lines for drying.
- Clothing can become contaminated by bacteria from residual scum forming inside machines which themselves can become damaged by the build-up of washing powder and clothing debris. The laundromat area should be regularly cleaned and serviced.
- Washing powder should be available at cost price in the dispensing machines.

- Public access to washing machines should be extended by providing a further facility in the community.
- Consideration of providing the option to private owners to have their machines repaired and serviced by a qualified person.

Action area: creating supportive environments
Decision-makers in the community had the opportunity to create an economic and political environment which supports access to hygiene products such as the purchase of essential hygiene items, providing a subsidy system to allow people to purchase these items and by extending access to the laundromat.

Action area: developing personal skills
The health promotion action area 'developing personal skills' provides opportunities for better access to information and education through the development of personal skills. Skill development increases the options available to people to exercise more control over their own health and environment. This can be facilitated in settings such as the local school or health centre and would involve technical skills training such as handwashing, defrosting and food storage and disposal of wastes. These are sensitive issues and would require learning through 'doing' and demonstrations rather than using a didactic approach.

Action area: reorienting health services
Health promotion is an inter-sectoral responsibility and the programme included collaboration between the Council of Elders, the school, the health centre, Environmental health Services and Housing Services. It is the role of the outside agent, the practitioners, to mediate and advocate on behalf of the community for these different authorities to come together to participate in the programme.

Case study 2: improving livelihoods in rural communities in Kyrgyzstan

Poverty alleviation has emerged as a central area of concern in rural development and has become inextricably linked to our understanding of rural livelihoods. This has given prominence to sustainable livelihoods as an objective, an approach and an analytical framework. The Sustainable Livelihoods for Livestock Programme (SLLP) in Kyrgyzstan, Central Asia, had identified strengthening community capacity as key to addressing the concern of improving the livelihoods of stakeholders. The SLLP (referred to as 'the Programme') is an initiative covering an estimated 28,500 people living in 14 pilot communities. The Programme has regional offices in the provinces of Chui, Osh and Talas, each with a resident team of national and international personnel to manage community-based activities. Regional staff provide a link between the communities and the Programme management unit in Bishkek, the capital city, which provides coordination and support.

The aim of the Programme was to:

- develop mechanisms for income generation from business and agricultural livestock production including cashmere fibre, handicrafts, honey, medicinal herbs and tourism;
- improve and promote access to support services;
- develop self-help capacities at community level and strengthen local agencies (Jones and Laverack 2003).

It is this last point, developing capacities at the community level, that is the community development focus of the Programme. It links closely to the concept of community empowerment by enabling people to take control of their lives, including their health. The primary role is to link material improvements in livelihoods to improvements in communities' abilities to take responsibility for their own health and future development. To assist this process, the Programme provides commercial credit, training, equipment, small-scale civil works and technical assistance.

The cultural context

Occupying 199,000 sq. km in the Tien Shan mountain range of Central Asia, west of China, what is now the Kyrgyz Republic came under Russian control in the late nineteenth century. The Soviet era largely reshaped the Kyrgyz economic and social institutions by forcibly shifting the population from transient pastoralists to sedentary collectivized agriculturalists or workers in state-planned factories. Independence in Kyrgyzstan in 1991 demonstrated that many Soviet-era institutions were unsustainable and this resulted in economic collapse and social crisis. Supported by the international community, the government rapidly embraced market-orientated reforms including widespread privatization, although the economy remains dominated by agriculture (Jones and Laverack 2003). The livelihoods of communities included in the Programme are based on a combination of agricultural activities such as wheat, potatoes and livestock rearing. Other local enterprises include cashmere fibre, handicrafts, bee products, medicinal herbs and tourism as a complement to, or substitute for, current sources of rural income.

The community empowerment approach

It was decided by all the stakeholders that there was insufficient time to complete a detailed and systematic approach to build community empowerment because of the imminent onset of winter. During the long winter months it is extremely difficult for community members to travel around the country, for example, to attend a workshop. Instead, it was decided by the stakeholders to prepare a contingent plan for community empowerment and then, the following summer, develop a more detailed strategy. The Programme held a workshop in Bishkek prior to the onset of winter and invited representatives from the communities to develop a plan to strengthen each of the nine empowerment domains as follows.

Participation. The Programme initially did not involve community representatives in decision-making and it was the outside agent who undertook the detailed planning. The main reason for this was to ensure that interventions were in place in time for reporting deadlines. Participation was compromised and community members were involved by simply attending meetings. As the Programme was implemented there were conscious changes in its operation to be more inclusive of the opinions of community members. For example, a number of discussion groups were facilitated to raise the concerns that the community would like to continue meeting around, to allow their representatives to take a greater role in decision-making in the Programme. Gaining trust and establishing common ground with community members were crucial to this process to involve people in the Programme in a much more meaningful way.

Leadership. Since independence in the Kyrgyz Republic, all types of organization (non-government, government and community-based) have tended to have weak procedures for governance, a limited vision of their aims and tasks, and lack a development strategy (Jones and Laverack 2003). The Programme would support community leadership in a number of practical ways including organizing exchange visits of the leaders of local craft associations to more advanced and established organizations elsewhere in the country. During these visits the leaders in the pilot communities could share experiences and ideas. The Programme also worked to establish good working relations with elected village leaders to enhance their standing with the communities in which they work. The Programme has worked toward building the accountability of these leaders – for example, in promoting transparent open accounting practices so that anyone can establish what was done, by whom and at what cost.

Organizational structures. A common characteristic of the communities with which the Programme worked was the existence of a large number of organizational structures including community councils, women and youth committees, farmers' cooperatives and water users' associations. Such 'public spaces' are slowly expanding in the Kyrgyz Republic and offer an opportunity for people to reflect and start questioning together, sharing experiences and developing solutions to address important issues in their lives. The role of the Programme has been to establish coordination mechanisms in each village to allow the representation of different groups to become involved in a wider range of decision-making exercises.

Supporting the coordination mechanisms are initiatives to provide resource centres as places where community organizations can conduct activities. Resource centres provide a facility, sometimes just a room, and a focal point in the community, where information can be easily accessed and contacts with outside links can be established. Many of the communities quickly recognized the value of the resource centre and it became intertwined with activities to generate income and raise new ideas in the community.

Problem assessment. The Programme assisted the pilot communities to develop new skills and competencies to carry out problem assessment. The communities then identified and prioritized the immediate (short-term) 'problems' in their lives as a focus for the planning of activities and for the raising of the resources necessary to support action. This can be assisted by an outside agent but for it to be an empowering experience it is the community that identifies the problem to be addressed.

Prioritization was necessary because the communities do not have the resources at their disposal to address all the domains as a part of the same strategy. The role of the Programme was to assist the community to gain access to resources (discussed later in 'Resource mobilization') and support services such as the supply of quality seed potatoes.

Asking why. This is distinct from the domain of problem assessment in that it encourages organizations to think beyond their own local concerns and to take a stronger position on broader issues. The Kyrgyz Republic, as a former part of the Soviet Union, has organizational structures at all levels that are inherently top-down and function within a rigid and controlled bureaucratic apparatus. Civil society is a relatively new concept for development in the country. Social and political conditions are not designed to facilitate critical awareness and, starved of outside information and influences, many communities develop an introspective nature, focusing only on their immediate needs and problems.

Rather than using an education approach the Programme decided to help community members in small 'working groups' to analyse why some people were poorer than others and what local, state and national actions might remedy their particular circumstances. Through these group discussions, facilitated by the Programme, individuals gradually became more critically aware of the broader issues of poverty in a process of discussion, reflection and action.

Resource mobilization. The community organizations started with limited resources. The people attending began to raise internal resources on a small scale through personal donations and contributions of local produce. The Programme then helped the organizations to obtain external funding through the development of their skills to prepare grant applications, organize meetings and keep accounts. The Programme resources were largely tied to conventional community development outcomes such as an increase in participation. The community members decided to identify ideas for funding that fell outside the conventional view of what were legitimate outcomes for a community development programme, such as the provision of a computer or facilities to be used by the village youth during the long winter months.

The Programme had other successes in helping communities to mobilize resources, in one case by offering matching funds to rehabilitate an irrigation pipe serving household plots. The Programme encouraged the community to mobilize approximately 60 per cent of the costs of materials, as well as supplying labour to install the replacement pipe. The community was able to raise these funds through a combination of individual contributions and allocations from the government budget (Jones and Laverack 2003).

Links to others. The Programme used strategies to develop partnerships with other local organizations involved in sustainable livelihoods. For example, by arranging 'exhibition days' to bring community organizations together in a mix of entertaining and informative activities to help establish contacts and share ideas. The Programme was also interested in linking the communities to local organizations including brokering ties with policy-makers. The position of the Programme was to support the points raised by community organizations, helping to legitimize their issues and advocating on their behalf in committees and technical meetings.

Outside agents. A programme in which an outside agent provides direct assistance to a community may serve to reinforce a sense of subordination and dependence on external sources among its members. This creates the practical dilemma of finding ways to assist community empowerment, in a programme context, without reinforcing dependency.

The first challenge for the Programme was to identify the communities' own sources of power (resources, decision-making authority, technical skills, local knowledge etc.). To do this the Programme assisted the community members to 'map' or identify the internal resources that they already had to help them build from a position of strength. Rather than begin their work from the perspective that people are, in general terms, 'relatively' economically and politically powerless, the Programme looked for, and worked from, areas in people's lives in which they were relatively powerful.

The second challenge for the Programme was to assist individuals to organize and mobilize themselves collectively through strengthening each of the empowerment domains. The third challenge was to support the creation of an adequate resource base for community action and to do this the

Programme acted as a link between the external resources and the community.

Programme management. Transferring responsibility for management is a long-term and ongoing process. As interventions linked to the short agricultural season came to a conclusion, the Programme actively involved community members in an assessment of achievements. Community 'working groups' and 'village resource centres' (referred to above) were actively used for this purpose. It was important that all sectors of the community knew what the Programme had contributed, what they had to contribute and that there was a common agreement on the outcomes. Community-based monitoring was seen as a means of drawing the communities further into the planning process. At the same time, knowledge gained since the beginning of the Programme was used to set out medium-term development perspectives for the pilot communities, creating a framework for focusing resources. This information was shared through community meetings and the detailed planning of interventions undertaken on the basis of an agreed work plan.

Over time, and as additional resources were obtained, the community took on more direct control of their activities including management, fundraising and liaison with other organizations and people. This was a reverse of the organizational circumstances seen at the beginning of the Programme when it was the outside agent who made most of the decisions.

The Programme has had to operate within an inherently top-down and rigid bureaucratic governmental apparatus. As a result it has been better able to support some empowerment domains over others. For example, success has been achieved in building empowered community organizations, strengthening links to other organizations and improving participation and resource mobilization. However, the development of trust between different Programme partners has been a slow process and enabling the pilot communities to understand the underlying causes of their poverty (critical awareness) is a long-term process that will extend beyond the Programme period.

Evaluating community empowerment

The Programme used the domains approach discussed in Chapter 5 and the spider-web configuration discussed in Chapter 6 to evaluate and visually represent community empowerment. The evaluation was carried out every six months over an 18-month period. Figure 8.1 shows the spider-web configuration for the Kopura bazaar community for the 6-month period between March and September. The spider-web shows that there was an improvement in the domains programme management, links to others, problem assessment, resource mobilization and local leadership. This was because the outside agency had embarked on initiatives to assist the community to identify its problems and then provide technical support for skills training in management and leadership. The Programme also supported a number of activities to develop partnerships with other communities, especially in the area of income generation, for example by using *hasars* (a form of traditional voluntary labour) to make and sell local crafts. There was no improvement in participation and critical awareness and a reduction in the domain village organizations or organizational structures. Critical awareness, as discussed earlier, is a difficult domain to develop in a context with a rigid and top-down bureaucratic apparatus. By introducing new ideas such as problem assessment and skills training, some community organizations decided to appoint new leaders and recruit new members. This resulted in conflict and reorganization and although it was a necessary step to improve community organizations it had the effect of temporarily reducing the evaluation of the domain during the first reevaluation.

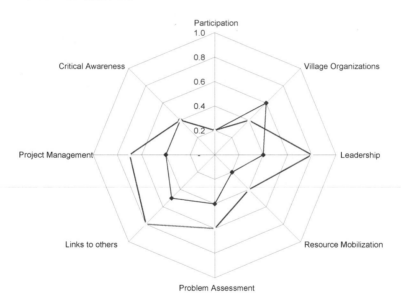

Figure 8.1 Spider-web for Kopuro bazaar community

Chapter 9 discusses the main lessons learnt in terms of building empowered communities and also three key contexts in which health promotion agencies, and the practitioners that they employ, can do this.

9 Building empowered communities

This final chapter brings together the central themes of the book and discusses the main lessons learnt regarding building empowered communities. The chapter also discusses three key perspectives, social, structural and radical, that will help health promotion agencies and practitioners to understand how community empowerment approaches are influenced.

Lessons learnt

The information provided in this book has shown that to be successful in building community empowerment the design of health promotion programmes should:

1 Address community concerns.
2 Build partnerships between the community, outside agencies and the practitioners that they employ.
3 Build community capacity to improve the knowledge, skills and competencies that enable communities to better address their concerns.
4 Evaluate their effectiveness and share ideas and visions with all stakeholders.

Addressing community concerns

A key lesson for empowering people is the preparedness of health promotion practice to identify, and support, those concerns 'close to the heart' of communities. There is sufficient evidence to show that if practitioners are not willing to address the concerns of communities then the programmes that they implement are much less likely to succeed. Who identifies the concern to be addressed and how this is taken forward is critical to building empowered communities. A key constraint to achieving this is the use of top-down approaches in health promotion programmes and the tension that this creates by not addressing community concerns through their design. In practice, a compromise often has to be met between the community concerns and what the implementing agency wants but may be restricted in achieving.

As discussed in Chapter 1, health promotion is most often delivered through top-down programmes controlled by government agencies or government-funded NGOs. It is government policy (and resources) that set the health promotion agenda and the difficulty begins when this does not meet community concerns. The reliance of health promotion on government funding has contributed to the dominance of top-down styles of programming. Health promotion practitioners are employed to design and deliver programmes that improve the health of individuals, groups and communities within the parameters set by government policy.

Even when those in the 'top' structures agree with those at the community level about the main concerns, the way in which the agenda is designed and implemented can result in the main issues not being addressed. For example, if you ask any reasonably poor person in any inner-city housing area what their leading concern is, 'drugs' would probably be among the top contenders. Relatively powerless groups share in common with more powerful groups the necessity to address the reality of this issue. Powerful groups, including politicians and health authorities, define the solution to the drug 'problem' in terms of more police, more social marketing programmes, more drug education courses, more drug rehabilitation programmes, and lots of anti-drug posters and pamphlets. Relatively powerless groups, including residents' associations and community groups, define the solution in terms of fear for safety, street violence, crime, poor street-lighting, unemployment and even poor housing repair. The solution of more police can create tensions because of racial issues and social marketing and health education do little to address the underlying social and structural causes of drug abuse (Labonte 1998).

Parallel examples also exist at the level of policy work in large organizations and institutions. Ronald Labonte (1998), a prominent health promotion philosopher, uses the example of one employer that initiated an internal workplace smoking ban as a 'test run' for a change in policy. The decision was based on advice from a health promotion practitioner and on requests from many employees. Negotiations took place between management, unions and the practitioner. Unsurprisingly, each stakeholder made a different claim to the issue. Management wanted to keep costs low and maintain labour peace, though they also had a concern for workers' well-being. Unions did not want worker solidarity split by pitting smokers against non-smokers, had a more general concern with overall indoor air quality and figured costs were a management concern. The practitioner simply wanted to eliminate all exposure to environmental tobacco smoke. After several months of negotiating to find the 'common ground', the issue was re-framed as one of 'no exposure to a known carcinogen', one which all three groups could support. Rather than opt for expensive, separately-vented smoking areas, all three stakeholder groups agreed to divert the funds to an overhaul of air ventilation systems and testing of other airborne toxins.

To begin to address community concerns the health promotion practitioner must build a partnership with their clients that is both supportive and non-controlling. The purpose is to facilitate the sharing of power in a way that involves the provision of both services and resources, at the request of the client.

Building partnerships

The role of the practitioner in a health promotion programme is initially concerned with providing leadership – for example, by setting up community groups and providing the enthusiasm and resources necessary to move participation forward. However, the expectation of this role can soon change to a position of a more 'equal' partnership between the practitioner and the community. Partnerships demonstrate the ability of the community to develop relationships with outside agents based on the recognition of mutual interests and respect. The partnership may involve an exchange of services, the pursuit of a joint venture based on a shared goal or an initiative to take action.

Many practitioners find it difficult to relinquish the control that they have over the design and implementation of a programme. Accepting the expertise of community knowledge, and sharing professional expertise so that community members can use it to build their own empowering capacities, can be an alien concept to health professionals. Angela Kilian, a British community organizer, studied the ability of a number of community health workers to reach this status in top-down health education groups. There was some resistance on the part of many of the participating women to taking control. This reflected the women's view of the group and the health worker as still belonging to the National Health Service. One could interpret their resistance to take control as a paradoxical exercise of control against an institution they may largely distrust. As this dynamic was slowly worked through, most groups managed some degree of shift in control over the activities, but one did not. This group was the only one led by a health professional who could not transcend the conditioned need to direct, judge and think always of group members in a paternalistic way (Kilian 1988).

Health promotion practitioners do have an important role in providing information (education and awareness activities), resources and technical assistance but this must support the concerns that have been identified by the community as being relevant and important to them. The role of the practitioner in a partnership is to assist people to build a greater sense of control in their lives. The first step towards taking more control can, for example, be through participating in small groups, receiving information that clarifies an issue or gaining new skills. The purpose is to allow individuals to better define, analyse and then to collectively act on issues of mutual concern.

Practitioners sometimes consciously do this by advising and educating their clients, by developing skills and connecting individuals to, for example, neighbourhood groups. But mostly practitioners are not aware of the importance of the role that they can play in empowering the individuals, groups and communities with which they work.

Building community capacity

Sometimes communities know what they want but do not know how to achieve it. In other instances, communities do not know what they want and are further constrained in identifying their concerns by internal conflict or a lack of understanding and skills. The practitioner has an important role to play, especially at the early stages of a programme, in providing the necessary support to help communities to identify and/or address their concerns. This is a temporary role and longer-term the practitioner should be working toward building the capacity of the community so that its members can take control of the programme.

The programme design should clearly define how it will build the capacity of the community from planning, through implementation, through management and evaluation. Without this focus the community can become dependent on the outside agent to provide support during the lifecycle of the programme without themselves building the necessary capacities. The way in which community capacity is addressed and defined is an important issue that is often overlooked in programming. It includes two key areas:

1   The capacity of the community to resolve its own concerns and the development of specific skills and competencies that contribute to their overall capacity. These skills may be used later in a variety of circumstances – for example, the organizational skills that are developed to address a local concern such as flooding may be used again to address the siting of a health centre. Building community capacity has a generic characteristic and is not limited to only one issue.
2   The capacity of the community to take more control of the programme involves skills development based on programme management such as financial management, report-writing and evaluation. These are skills and capacities that the community can use when it is involved in programme management.

The concept of parallel tracking, discussed in Chapter 4, and the domains approach discussed in Chapter 5, are designed to be used in conjunction with one another as a systematic means to help communities to build their capacity, centred on their concerns in a programme context.

The provision of resources and technical support is the basis of partner-ships developing between the outside agent and the community. The key point here is to provide the appropriate level of support at the request of the community. This means that the outside agent should not commit all the resources at the planning stage of the programme. This is because new re-source inputs will be identified as the strategic plan of the community is developed. To meet this demand the outside agent should be flexible in the type of resources that they are prepared to provide to support the community.

In a programme context, resources are often designated to a specific budget category – for example, travel costs, training and equipment. How-ever, the resources requested by the community may not fit neatly into one of these categories. For example, in many South Pacific cultures it is customary for meetings to begin with a formal ceremony. This involves introductory speeches by the guests and senior members of the group and the acceptance and drinking of *kava*. Katz (1993) points out that in Fiji the *sevusevu* must initiate all major meetings because it is the cultural way of asking the an-cestral gods, the *Vu*, for their permission and blessing to proceed. This cere-mony must be respected and although the guest presents *kava* to another person it is actually being received by the *Vu* who stand behind the human participants. The drinking of *kava* in formal settings also has another social purpose. Because of its mild psychoactive and soporific effect it helps to mellow the atmosphere and encourages discussion. *Kava* drinking provides the opportunity to bring people together to identify and resolve their con-cerns but it would be difficult to justify the purchase of this product from the budget of a health promotion programme!

There are other activities that are difficult to justify as being strictly health promotion but that nonetheless build the social dimension of com-munities through a sense of belonging, connectedness and personal re-lationships. For example, traditional singing and dancing, a sporting event, a barbeque or the sale of food and locally-made crafts. In addition to raising internal resources these activities create a sense of community, bringing dif-ferent groups and clans together and bonding them through their own tra-ditional customs and rituals. The flexibility of resource allocation should allow these types of activities so as to build community empowerment.

Evaluating and sharing ideas and visions

The need for dialogue, the free flow of information and open communication between the practitioner and their clients is essential for empowerment. To avoid misunderstandings the expectations must be clearly defined, docu-mented, shared and discussed. The need for the free and equitable flow of information has also been identified as an important element in the process of community empowerment by other authors, who highlight inter-agency collaboration and effective communication (MaCallan and Narayan 1994) and a dialogue between the community organization and the individual community members (Speer and Hughey 1995).

One purpose of evaluation is to empower people by addressing their concerns. In practice, this means providing people with the information that they need to make informed decisions and to plan strategies to improve their lives and health. However, the sharing of information from one person to others, even when everyone has an equal sense of ownership, can present a challenge. It is crucial that this information is in a format that can be understood by community members as well as practitioners.

Visual representation provides a practical way to share the analysis and interpretation of the measurement of empowerment with all stakeholders. Visual representation also allows information to be compared over a specific timeframe, between the different components within a programme and between programmes. Visual representations do not have to use text and are therefore useful in a cross-cultural perspective or when stakeholders are not literate. The use of one visual representation, the spider-web configuration, is discussed in different cultural contexts in Chapter 6.

As discussed in Chapter 1, the key to empowering communities is transforming unequal power relationships which are indicative of our society and working practices. Next, I discuss three different perspectives in which health promotion practitioners and the agencies that employ them can work with others to build community empowerment: social, structural and radical.

The social perspective

The social perspective describes the network of support through which people interact to organize and mobilize themselves. Social networks have been associated with improvements in health – for example, a lower total mortality by reducing deaths from cardiovascular disease and suicide (Kawachi *et al.* 1996; Rosengren *et al.* 2004). Social networks and social support are developed through a process of interaction, as discussed in Chapter 2, at the individual, group and community levels. To address the inequalities in health individuals have a better chance of success if they can act collectively. It is through collective action that people can increase their access to resources, influence decisions and build support through wider participation. It is governments that create the policies and regulations that are responsible for the distribution of power that can lead to inequalities in health. By increasing their membership and resource base, communities are better able to have an influence both on civil society and on government structures. They do this by gaining greater control over the distribution of power that affects their lives and health.

In most democratic countries, community empowerment is used to influence public, economic and regulatory policies. They are influenced through the legitimate actions of individuals and sometimes through non-legitimate means, discussed later in the radical perspective. This is a process that can be facilitated by practitioners. In practice, it means helping individuals to make decisions and to participate in groups and organizations that share their concerns. Participation can often be the first step for many individuals toward collective action and an increase in their skills through working with others. However, individuals, groups and communities only begin to become fully empowered when they address the social and political causes of powerlessness that influence their lives.

In response to community demands governments often place the onus of responsibility on individuals, groups and communities. An example of this is government-sponsored awareness campaigns to provide information to create an 'informed choice'. This is a secure approach because it commits those in authority to only provide information, usually in a one-way direction by using the mass media, to inform people or to 'engage' them in passive forms of participation. However, communities must be careful because their patronage in these programmes can result in their right to take action against those in power being compromised. Participation can allow those who hold power to claim that all sides were considered while only a few benefit, thus helping to maintain the status quo.

An empowering approach to health promotion goes much further than this. Empowerment is used to influence public, economic and regulatory policies through the legitimate actions of people in 'communities of interest' who use their decision-making power – for example, voting at a local or national election or by placing their name on a petition. Communities can take other indirect actions such as registering a complaint to a local authority and writing a letter to their Member of Parliament or a local newspaper about their concerns. People, individually or collectively, also have other and more direct means to influence government policy to make the necessary changes to improve their lives and health – for example, they can take legal action, fund a publicity campaign, lobby, demonstrate and carry out civil protests against those they feel are the cause of their powerlessness.

Communities can be assisted in this process by providing them with the necessary information or skills to undertake action – for example, a list of other concerned groups, access to the internet and relevant websites, leadership training and fundraising skills.

The structural perspective

The structural perspective is that of the state, the government and those in authority who hold political and economic power over others. The structural perspective includes the means of governing people and is itself dependent on 'expert' systems of knowledge and truths as a means by which to regulate and manage individuals. Its organizational structure is most visible as the bureaucracies of institutions and large organizations and the positions of control that they create with specialist and formally-defined duties. For example, in many countries the head of the Department of Health exerts considerable influence over health policy development which permeates 'down' to the wider community of health authorities, trusts, care groups, advisory bodies and practitioners. The structural perspective is therefore central to setting the policies and rules that influence our health.

As discussed in Chapter 4, health promotion is a part of the structural perspective. An empowering health promotion practice aims to bring about changes in the social and political distribution of power in favour of those that do not have it and that struggle to gain it. To do this health promotion engages its clients in political activities to enable them to gain better access to decisions and resources that affect their lives. This can mean collectively working toward a change in the law such as a local bylaw to prohibit dog-walking on beaches to protect public health; or collectively working toward broader policy change such as providing women with access to the most effective drugs to treat breast cancer; or collective action to change the normative values held by society such as publicly and collectively shaming those who commit domestic violence. For example, anecdotal reports of pot- or bottle-banging were gathered by patrons at a local pub in Thembisa, South Africa upon witnessing a man physically abusing his girlfriend. Similarly, there were unconfirmed reports of pot-banging taking place in Khayelitsha, South Africa over the evaluation period of an intervention undertaken by Soul City and the National Network on Violence Against Women. These stories depicted the community's shift from 'silent collusion' with domestic violence to active opposition. This activity was introduced in a story broadcast as part of a nationwide intervention and had not been heard of in South Africa previously (Soul City 4 2001).

The structural perspective often undertakes a process of 'consultation' with communities to try and understand what people want. This can sometimes unrealistically raise community expectations and create a demand for further government support. Unless those in authority are committed to move forward with what people really want it runs the real risk of contributing to their sense of powerlessness. What those in power are saying is, 'We have consulted with you and hear what you are saying but we have a more important agenda than yours'. Community needs do not always match government agendas. For example, lifestyle interventions aimed at increasing exercise or changing diet may seem unimportant to people who suffer mental ill health, are unemployed, poor or live in an area of high crime. These people have different priorities and may not think about the consequences of everyday choices such as exercise and diet even if they had the resources to make such lifestyle changes possible.

To move forward with what people want, the structural perspective must have the mechanisms in place to facilitate the necessary changes through, for example, policy and legislation to create supportive environments that make the 'healthy choice the easier choice'. Programmes that are more empowering include those aimed at 'early education for all' such as neighbourhood nurseries. For example, the Sure Start programme in the UK provides free part-time education for 3- to 4-year-olds. The programme makes child care more accessible, better quality, more affordable and provides information to parents about services offered. The programme establishes child care facilities at subsidized rates and in disadvantaged areas to offer poor families early education, health and family support (Department of Education 2006).

Transforming inequalities in the distribution of power in the long term requires political action on issues such as the causes of poverty through policies that influence welfare services, housing, transport policy and community health services. The structural perspective has an important role in promoting social justice and equality, and addressing the determinants of health.

The structural perspective and the determinants of health

To address the determinants of health governments must take a long-term approach to redress the causes of social and economic inequality such as unemployment. Governments can have a significant impact on the health and lives of people through policies and legislation. These policies include:

- improving the standards of teaching and resource allocation in schools;
- minimum wage and working hours;
- creating better opportunities to find work;
- vocational and skills training;
- preventive services and the education of mothers about child care;
- better access to affordable child care facilities;
- building community support and social interaction;
- better access to public transport;
- better access to exercise facilities such as cycle paths (Wilkinson 2003).

Governments also need to engage health promotion agencies and their clients in social and political action. While health promotion agencies cannot be expected to change these long-term goals by themselves they do have a crucial role to play in the redistribution of power, in supporting government policy and in their control over decisions and resources that influence people's health. In particular, there are two areas of importance in which they have a role:

1   Practitioners are involved in influencing policies and practices which affect health, from national down to the community level – for example, through their 'expert' power in meetings and committees. In order to influence policy and practice, practitioners need to have a better understanding of the meaning of power, the relationships with their clients and how these can be appropriately acted upon by different professional groups.

2   In many countries the process of collective action is used to influence social and political changes through regulatory policies. These changes are achieved through the legitimate action of individuals who use their decision-making power, for example, by taking legal action against those in power. Practitioners, in their day-to-day work with individuals and groups, can help their clients to use their six bases of power-over (discussed in Chapter 1) to have a greater influence over political and economic policy that in turn influences the determinants of health. To be more empowering in their work, practitioners need to have a clear understanding of the influence that they can have on the process of community empowerment (Laverack 2005).

The role of the practitioner is to involve individuals, groups and communities who have shared concerns so that they can identify solutions and actions to address the issues. Participation is often the first step by which governments can help people to become involved in collective action and from which they can then work towards empowerment. This step is facilitated by introducing people to networks of other concerned individuals, support groups and community-based organizations. Participation in groups, organizations and communities builds their level of social support and interaction – for example, by sharing problems people are better able to cope with stressful events because this helps them to see the world as being more manageable and meaningful (Wilkinson 1996; Geyer 1997). Social support is generally accepted as an important determinant of health and provides a favourable environment in which a dialogue, problem identification and resolution can take place and in turn can lead to empowerment (Wallerstein 1992).

Communities consist of competing power relations between individuals and between and within groups. The delivery of inputs within a health promotion programme context does not guarantee that those with the power over others, such as leaders, will choose to use their control of the limited resources to benefit individuals and groups that suffer the worst health inequalities. Governments must be prepared to reorientate professional practice to specifically help individuals, groups and communities to gain power.

Helping individuals to gain power involves building their power from within and helping them to participate in 'interest' groups and self-help groups. Individuals must have the self-confidence to participate and interact in a group setting in such a way as to make their opinions and concerns count. People achieve this through the gradual development of social networks, the mobilizing of resources and improving skills and capacities towards achieving their goals. Agencies can help individuals to gain more power by giving advice, connecting them with others and by sharing power with their clients in a way that involves the provision of both services and resources.

The structural perspective can play an important role in shaping and defining what is important – for example, it can endorse the concerns of less powerful interest groups and communities and this gives those concerns more professional and political credibility that can lead to funding opportunities. Helping groups and communities to gain power is a process of building skills, competencies and capacities that can be supported as part of the everyday work of practitioners. Community empowerment can be enhanced by practitioners who help to develop stronger organizational structures and broader networks. The development of interest groups into larger community organizations is crucial for them to make the transition to a broader network of alliances. It is through these partnerships that organizations are able to gain greater support and resources to achieve a favourable solution for their particular concerns. Community organizations include youth groups and community-based committees, cooperatives and associations. These are the organizational elements in which people come together in order to socialize and to address their broader concerns. Community organizations are not only larger than small mutual groups, they also have an established structure, more functional leadership, the ability to better organize their members to mobilize resources and to gain the skills that are necessary to allow small groups to make the transition to partnerships and alliances. These skills include planning and strategy development, management of time, team-building, networking, negotiation, fundraising, marketing, managing publicity and proposal-writing. Community organizations focus outwards to the environment that creates their needs in the first place, or offers the means of resolving them. Once the community has become more critically aware of the underlying causes of its powerlessness it can take the necessary steps to develop actions to redress the situation and try and gain more power (Laverack 2005: 69).

The structural perspective can help communities to become more critically reflective on their own circumstances. But to be effective in influencing 'higher level' policy decision-making, community organizations need to link with others sharing similar concerns. The purpose of establishing partnerships is to allow community organizations to grow beyond their own local concerns and to take a stronger position on broader issues, through networking and resource mobilization, such as health services delivery, a minimum wage and improved working conditions.

The important role of health promotion agencies can be constrained by the bureaucratic nature of the structural perspective. Health promotion agencies and practitioners who are largely employed by governments work with individuals, groups and communities in civil society to promote their health and well-being. This can create a problematic relationship between the state and civil society and to bridge the gap health promotion practice must be flexible in the way it designs, delivers and evaluates its programmes. Bureaucratic settings often remain governed by traditional ways of thinking and acting, ways which inhibit the effective inclusion of empowering approaches. The dominance of top-down approaches and rigid funding cycles and the use of manipulative methods to influence the way people behave and what they know can constrain empowerment. The use of parallel tracking and the inclusion of empowerment goals in top-down programming, discussed in Chapter 4, are practical examples of how practitioners can address these constraints.

The radical perspective

The increase in political instability and forms of government dominated by elite group interests can lead to the oppression of community-based interaction including empowerment. These circumstances can lead to an atmosphere in which individuals, groups and communities strive to seize power from those in authority. The disruption they create and the level of public support that they can generate become key tactics to gain power. This is the radical perspective. It is a limited option but as Frances Piven and Richard Cloward (1977), two early commentators on poor people's movements, point out, historically the radical perspective has given rise to examples of dramatic social and political change resulting from community action such as the protests and riots among the lower classes over rent increases in the USA during the middle years of the twentieth century. In oppressive social and political circumstances it is often the most effective means of utilizing the limited resources available to very marginalized communities of interest.

A broad example of this can be seen in the environment movement. To gain a seat in the corporate-government boardrooms where environmental policies were being formed, this movement engaged in direct action campaigns that blocked effluent pipes, stopped polluting activities or prevented logging. Only when the day-to-day exercise of power-over by elite groups is disrupted by such protest are the conditions for negotiated partnerships or empowering approaches to programmes and policy change created. Moreover, such disruptions may continue to be required to prevent elite groups from co-opting those with whom they negotiate, or turning their back on partnerships once the opposition has been placated. Thus, the environmental movement today, like many other social movements, has groups that sit around the table in partnership with government and corporate leaders (Labonte 1990).

But not all partnerships are equal. Barbara Gray (1989), a seminal writer on interorganizational collaboration, comments that often 'weaker' partners must first develop their capacities, usually through community empowerment, before the conditions for an equitable partnership between the state and civil society can exist. One of the key conditions for partnerships is that no one party has the power to act unilaterally. It is precisely under oppressive governance systems that unilateral power exists. But even in democratic systems a few stakeholders often have monopoly power around certain issues. Barbara Gray argues that effective partnerships around these issues can only occur after successful political struggles and community mobilizing efforts have given greater 'power' or voice to less powerful stakeholders.

Moving beyond conflict to partnerships, then, is only possible after less powerful groups have created, through political conflict, their identity as legitimate stakeholders, their ability to mobilize resources and their ability to prevent the unilateral actions of more powerful stakeholders. The environment movement therefore has groups that mobilize local indignation around specific environmental incidents. It also has groups that continue with direct action to keep the pressure on elite stakeholders to negotiate in good faith.

In the radical perspective, practitioners have the option of exercising their own voices as citizens – for example, through their participation in social movements such as Greenpeace, to support their agenda. In the same way, practitioners can act as organized groups of professionals to support the actions of communities of interest who they believe will benefit public health or who suffer from inequalities in power. They can endorse the concerns of these less powerful groups to provide some professional credibility – for example, the support of the medical profession against smoking has given credibility to this political lobby and in the Republic of Ireland and Scotland this has contributed to a nationwide ban on smoking in public places because of the associated health risks of passive smoking.

The ultra-radical

In health promotion, community empowerment is viewed as a process of collective action toward positive changes in favour of those seeking to gain more control in their lives. But in the twenty-first century there has been a growth in concern among civil society and those in political power about another form of community empowerment: terrorism. The process by which very different communities of interest seek to gain power from those who hold it provides a basic logic which has historically been shown to be similar. For example, the collective action of slaves in the Servile wars in Italy between 135–71 BC (Fast 1952), mass revolts leading to social and political changes in Haiti and San Domingo between 1791 and 1803 (James 1980), accounts of collective empowerment among the lower classes in the USA during the mid-twentieth century (Piven and Cloward 1977) and the political influence of ordinary people who helped end the apartheid period in South Africa in the latter years of the twentieth century (Hildebrandt 1996).

In the present-day context, parents concerned about, for example, the safety of their children in school playgrounds undergo the same process of social and organizational development as, for example, marginalized groups who are outraged by the occupation of their country by a foreign force. Both examples are concerned with the distribution of power and both have the aim of bringing about social and political change in favour of a community of interest. The first example is about the struggle for power over resources and decisions regarding the health and safety of children. The second is about the struggle for power over resources and decisions for the security of people both within and outside a particular geographical location. Crucially, both involve a process or continuum that is influenced by the nine empowerment domains. The difference lies in the means and methods that a community of interest is prepared to use to change the distribution of power.

Ordinary citizens collectively use participation, organizational structures, resource mobilization and local leaders to legitimately gain access to resources and decisions. They use methods such as voting, demonstrating and legal action and may even resort to tactics such as strike action, aggressive publicity campaigns or public protests against those in power. But in situations where people feel that social justice in society does not exist and when they lose their basic rights (e.g. to protest or to a fair voting and legal system), they must use the only significant resource they have: the capacity to cause trouble. The tactics they use are riots, revolts, insurgency and violence or the threat of violence. The terror they create and the reaction of those in power become the basis for political influence. This is a risky option and the gamble is that it will give rise to dramatic social and political change. In such instances of ultra-radical action the community of interest must maximize its efforts to succeed and push for full concessions in return for a cessation of the disruption.

This can be costly but in circumstances in which people believe they have nothing to lose – for example, when they have no employment, no property or no hope for the future, then it is a logical 'make or break' option. It is a desperate solution but the most effective means of utilizing the limited resources available (Piven and Cloward 1977). These communities of interest also embark on a process that includes participation, strengthening of organizational structures, improving leadership and resource mobilization. The communities develop networks which share resources and this has especially been the case with international terrorist organizations who share expertise, personnel and information. For example, guns stolen from a US army base in Germany were subsequently used by Japanese terrorist organizations (Russell *et al.* 1979). The members are also highly motivated and share common beliefs and concerns but ultimately they use tactics based on coordinated attacks that are often indiscriminate and target innocent people not involved in the issue, with a disregard for human life. Community empowerment can have a negative impact on people's lives when they are affected by a process that can promote violence and fear.

Outside agents can choose to use approaches that employ the nine empowerment domains to build empowered communities. The purpose is to give people more control over their lives and to have a positive impact on their health and its determinants. Conversely, the empowerment domains could also be used by an outside agent to undermine community-based interaction to promote the opposite of power: powerlessness. This could be achieved by using strategies that, for example, reduce participation, weaken leadership, destroy organizational structures, minimize resource mobilization, destabilize partnerships and links with others, confuse needs assessment and promote the power-over of the outside agent. We live in a world in which access to resources and decisions is limited and competing communities of interest must struggle to gain control. This includes the competition between those groups that strive to bring about social and political change through violence. As outside agents, we may have to carefully consider with whom and how we work with others to help them gain power.

This book has explained how health promotion agencies, and the practitioners that they employ, can work with communities to help them to gain more control over their lives by helping them to use whatever *legitimate* means they have available. Not all communities want to be or can be helped and not all practitioners want to help empower their clients. Nevertheless, health promotion, in both principle and practice, has a role to facilitate the empowerment of others. I have argued that this is an achievable and worthwhile use of health promotion resources.

Bibliography

Alinsky, S.D. (1972) *Rules For Radicals: A Practical Primer for Realistic Radicals*. New York: Vintage Books.

Arnstein, S.R. (1969) A ladder of citizen participation, *Journal of the American Institute of Planners*, July: 216–23.

Baggott, R. (2000) *Public Health: Policy and Politics*. London: St. Martin's Press, LLC.

Bailey, L. (1991) Being accountable: issues in community development and health work, in *Roots and Branches*, papers from the OU/HEA 1990 Winter School on Community Development and Health.

Balcazar, F.E. and Suarez-Balcazar, Y. (1996) *A Conceptual Model of Community Participation in Child Survival Programs*. Washington, DC: USAID.

Barnes, M. (2002) User movements, community development and health promotion, in L. Adams, M. Amos and J. Munro (eds) (2002) *Promoting Health: Politics and Practice*. London: Sage.

Barr, A. (1995) Empowering communities-beyond fashionable rhetoric? Some reflections on Scottish experience, *Community Development Journal*, 30(2): 121–32.

Bell-Woodward, G., Chad, K., Labonte, R. and Martin, L. (2005) Community capacity assessment of an active living health promotion program: 'saskatoon in motion'. University of Saskatchewan (unpublished).

Bjaras, G., Haglund, B.J.A. and Rifkin, S. (1991) A new approach to community participation evaluation, *Health Promotion International*, 6(3): 1999–206.

Blair, D. and Bernard, J.R.L. (eds) (1998) *Macquarie Pocket Dictionary*. Sydney: Jacaranda Wiley.

Bopp, M., Germann, K., Bopp, J., Littlejohns, L.B. and Smith, N. (1999) *Evaluating Community Capacity for Change*. Calgary: Four Worlds Development.

Boutilier, M. (1993) *The Effectiveness of Community Action in Health Promotion: A Research Perspective*. Toronto: University of Toronto.

Braithwaite, R.L., Bianchi, C. and Taylor, S.E. (1994) Ethnographic approach to community organisation and health empowerment, *Health Empowerment*, 21(3): 407–16.

Bratt, J.H., Weaver, M.A., Foreit, J., De Vargas, T. and Janowitz, B. (2002) The impact of price changes on demand for family planning and reproductive health services in Ecuador, *Health Policy and Planning*, 17(3): 281–7.

Brehm, J. and Rahn, W. (1997) Individual-level evidence for the causes and consequences of social capital, *American Journal of Political Science*, 41: 999–1023.

Britten, N. (1995) Qualitative interviews in medical research, *British Medical Journal*, 311: 251–3.

Brunner, E. (1996) The social and biological basis of cardiovascular disease in office workers, in D. Blane, E. Brunner and R. Wilkinson (eds) *Health and Social Organisation: Towards a Health Policy for the 21st Century*. New York: Routledge.

Bryman, A. (1992) *Quantity and Quality in Social Research.* London: Routledge.

Butterfoss, F.D., Goodman, R.M. and Wandersman, A. (1996) Community coalitions for prevention and health promotion: factors predicting satisfaction, participation and planning, *Health Education Quarterly*, 23(1): 65–79.

Carapetis, J.R., Johnston, F., Nadjamerrek,, J. and Kairupan, J. (1995) Skin sores in Aboriginal children, *Journal of Paediatrics and Child Health*, 31: 563.

Carr, A. (2000) *Community Project Workers Scheme Crime Prevention Projects: Evaluation Report.* Wellington: Community Development Group. Department of Internal Affairs. Government of New Zealand.

Cass, A., Lowell, A., Christie, M., Snelling, P.L., Flack, M., Marrnganyin, B. and Brown, I. (2002) Sharing the true stories: improving communication between Aboriginal patients and health care workers, *The Medical Journal of Australia*, 176(10): 466–70.

CDC/ATSDR, Committee on Community Engagement (1997) *Principles of Community Engagement*. Atlanta, GA: 62–3.

Clegg, S.R. (1989) *Frameworks of Power*. London: Sage.

Cohen, D.R. and Henderson, J.B. (1991) *Health, Prevention and Economics*. Oxford: Oxford University Press.

Coleman, P.T. (2000) Power and conflict, in M. Deutsch and P.T. Coleman (eds) *The Handbook of Conflict Resolution: Theory and Practice*. San Francisco: Jossey-Bass.

Constantino-David, K. (1995) Community organising in the Philippines: the experience of development NGOs, in G. Craig and M. Mayo (eds) (1995) *A Reader in Participation and Development*. London: Zed books.

Conway, K. (2002) Booze and beach bans: turning the tide through community action in New Zealand, *Health Promotion International*, 17(2): 171–7.

Cracknell, B.E. (1996) Evaluating development aid, *Evaluation*, 2(1): 23–33.

Department of Education (2006) *Welcome to Sure Start*. London: Department of Education, www.surestart.gov.uk.

Earle, L., Fozilhujaev, B., Tashbaeva, C. and Djamankulova, K. (2004) Community development in Kazakhstan, Kyrgyzstan and Uzbekistan, occasional paper no. 40. Oxford: INTRAC.

Eng, E. and Parker, E. (1994) Measuring community competence in the Mississippi Delta: the interface between programme evaluation and empowerment, *Health Education Quarterly*, 21(2): 199–220.

Everson, S.A., Lynch, J.W., Chesney, M.A., Kaplan, G.A., Goldberg, D.E., Shade, S.B., Cohen, R.D., Salonen, R. and Salonen, J.T. (1997) Interaction of workplace demands and cardiovascular reactivity in progression of carotid atherosclerosis: population-based study, *British Medical Journal*, 314: 553–8.

Ewles, L. and Simnett, I. (2003) *Promoting Health: A Practical Guide,* 5th edn. London: Bailliere Tindall.

Fast, H. (1952) *Spartacus.* London: Bantam Books.

Fetterman, D.M., Kaftarian, S.J. and Wandersman, A. (eds) (1996) *Empowerment Evaluation: Knowledge and Tools for Self-Assessment & Accountability.* Thousand Oaks, CA: Sage.

Freire, P. (1973) *Education for Critical Consciousness.* New York: Seabury Press.

Geyer, S. (1997) Some conceptual considerations on the sense of coherence, *Social Science Medicine*, 44(12): 1771–9.

Gibbon, M. (1999) Meetings with meaning: health dynamics in rural Nepal, unpublished Ph.D. thesis, South Bank University, London.

Gibbon, M., Labonte, R. and Laverack, G. (2002) Evaluating community capacity, *Health and Social Care in the Community*, 10(6): 485–91.

Goodman, R.M., Speers, M.A., McLeroy, K., Fawcett, S., Kegler, M., Parker, E., Rathgeb Smith, S., Sterling, T.D. and Wallerstein, N. (1998) Identifying and defining the dimensions of community capacity to provide a basis for measurement, *Health Education & Behavior*, 25(3): 258–78.

Gordon, G. (1995) Participation, empowerment and sexual health in Africa, in G. Craig, G. and M. Mayo (eds) (1995) *Community Empowerment: A Reader in Participation and Development.* London: Zed Books.

Gray, B. (1989) *Collaborating: Finding Common Ground for Multiparty Problems.* San Francisco: Jossey-Bass.

Green, L. and Kreuter, M. (1991) *Health Promotion Planning: An Educational and Environmental Approach.* Toronto: Mayfield Publishing.

Guba, E.G. (1990) *The Paradigm Dialog.* London: Sage.

Guba, E.G. and Lincoln, Y.S. (1989) *Fourth Generation Evaluation.* Newbury Park, CA: Sage.

Hashagen, S. (2002) *Models of Community Engagement.* Edinburgh: Scottish Community Development Centre.

Hauritz, M., Homel, R., Townsley, M., Burrows, T. and McIlwain, G. (1998) *An Evaluation of the Local Government Safety Actions Projects in Cairns, Townsville and Mackay.* Report to the Queensland Department of Health and the Criminology Research Council. Queensland: Griffith University and Queensland Department of Health.

Havemann, K. (2006) Effective participation in health development: why, who and how? Unpublished Ph.D. thesis, University of London.

Hawe, P., King, L., Noort, M., Jordens, C. and Lloyd, B. (2000) *Indicators to Help with Capacity-building in Health Promotion.* Sydney: Australian Centre for Health Promotion/NSW Health.

Hildebrandt, E. (1996) Building community participation in health care: a model and example from South Africa, *Image: Journal of Nursing Scholarship*, 28(2): 155–9.

Holder, H., Saltz, R., Grube, J., Voas, R., Gruenewald, P. and Treno, A. (1997) A community prevention trial to reduce alcohol involved accidental injury and death: overview, *Addiction*, 92: S155–71.

Homel, R., Hauritz, M., Wortley, R., McIlwain, G. and Carvolth, R. (1997) Preventing alcohol-related crime through community action: the Surfers Paradise Safety Action Project, *Crime Prevention Studies*, 7: 35–90.

IRED (1997) *People's Empowerment: Grassroots Experiences in Africa, Asia and Latin America*. Rome: IRED-NORD.

Israel, B.A., Checkoway, B., Schultz, A. and Zimmerman, M. (1994) Health education and community empowerment: conceptualizing and measuring perceptions of individual, organisational and community control, *Health Education Quarterly*, 21(2): 149–70.

Jackson, T., Mitchell, S. and Wright, M. (1989) The community development continuum, *Community Health Studies*, 8(1): 66–73.

James, C. (1980) *The Black Jacobins: Toussaint L'overture and the San Domingo Revolution*. London: Allison & Busby.

James, C. (1995) *Empowering Communities in the Development Process: Participatory Rural Appraisal as an Approach*. Bristol: University of Bristol.

Jones, A. and Laverack, G. (2003) *Building Capable Communities within a Sustainable Livelihoods Approach: Experiences from Central Asia*, www.livelihoods.org.

Jones, L. and Sidell, M. (eds) (1997) *The Challenge of Promoting Health: Exploration and Action*. London: Macmillan.

Jones, L., Sidell, M. and Douglas, J. (eds) (2002) *The Challenge of Promoting Health: Exploration and Action*, 2nd edn. London: Macmillan.

Katz, R. (1993) *The Straight Path: A Story of Healing and Transformation in Fiji*. New York: Addison-Wesley.

Kawachi, I., Colditz, G.A., Ascherio, A., Rimm, E.B., Giovannucci, E., Stampfer, M.J. and Willett, W.C. (1996) A prospective study of social networks in relation to total mortality and cardiovascular disease in men in the USA, *Journal of Epidemiology and Community Health*, 50: 245–51.

Kieffer, C.H. (1984) Citizen empowerment: a development perspective, *Prevention in Human Services*, 3: 9–36.

Kilian, A. (1988) Conscientisation: an empowering, nonformal education approach for community health workers, *Community Health Journal*, 23(2): 117–23.

Kitzinger, J. (1995) Introducing focus groups, *British Medical Journal*, 311: 299–302.

Korsching, P.F. and Borich, T.O. (1997) Facilitating cluster communities: lessons from the Iowa experience, *Community Development Journal*, 32(4): 342–53.

Kukuruzovic, R., Haase, A., Dunn, K., Bright, A. and Brewster, D.R. (1999) Intestinal permeability and diarrhoeal disease in Aboriginal Australians, *Archives for Diseases of Children*, 81: 304–8.

Kumpfer, K., Turner, C., Hopkins, R. and Librett, J. (1993) Leadership and team effectiveness in community coalitions for the prevention of alcohol and other drug abuse, *Health Education Research, Theory and Practice*, 8(3): 359–74.

Labonte, R. (1990) Empowerment: notes on professional and community dimensions, *Canadian Review of Social Policy*, (26): 64–75.

Labonte, R. (1993) *Health Promotion and Empowerment: Practice Frameworks*. Toronto: University of Toronto.

Labonte, R. (1994) Health promotion and empowerment: reflections on professional practice, *Health Education Quarterly*, 21(2): 253–68.

Labonte, R. (1996) Community development in the public health sector: the possibilities of an empowering relationship between the state and civil society, Ph.D. thesis, York University, Toronto.

Labonte, R. (1998) *A Community Development Approach to Health Promotion: A Background Paper on Practice Tensions, Strategic Models and Accountability Requirements for Health Authority Work on the Broad Determinants of Health*. Edinburgh: Health Education Board for Scotland.

Labonte, R. and Laverack, G. (2001) Capacity-building in health promotion, part 1: for whom and for what purpose? *Critical Public Health*, 11(2): 111–28.

Labonte, R. and Robertson, A. (1996) Delivering the goods, showing our stuff: the case for a constructivist paradigm for health promotion and research, *Health Education Quarterly*, 23(4): 431–47.

Laverack, G. (1998) The concept of empowerment in a traditional Fijian context, *Journal of Community Health and Clinical Medicine for the Pacific*, 5(1):26–9.

Laverack, G. (1999) Addressing the contradiction between discourse and practice in health promotion, unpublished Ph.D. thesis, Deakin University, Melbourne.

Laverack, G. (2000) *Health and Housing Repair in a Rural Community in the Northern Territory of Australia*. North Darwin, Australia: Territory Health Services.

Laverack, G. (2001) An identification and interpretation of the organizational aspects of community empowerment, *Community Development Journal*, 36(2): 40–52.

Laverack, G. (2003) Building capable communities: experiences in a rural Fijian context, *Health Promotion International*, 18(2): 99–106.

Laverack, G. (2004) *Health Promotion Practice: Power and Empowerment*. London: Sage.

Laverack, G. (2005) *Public Health: Power, Empowerment and Professional Practice*. London: Palgrave Macmillan.

Laverack, G. (2006a) Using a 'domains' approach to build community empowerment, *Community Development Journal*, 41(1): 4–12.

Laverack, G. (2006b) Improving health outcomes through community empowerment: a review of the literature, *Journal of Health Population and Nutrition*, 24(1): 113–20.

Laverack, G. (2006c) Evaluating community capacity: visual representation and interpretation, *Community Development Journal*, 41(3): 266–76.

Laverack, G. and Brown, K.M. (2003) Qualitative research in a cross-cultural context: Fijian experiences, *Qualitative Health Research*, 13(3): 1–10.

Laverack, G. and Dao, H.D. (2003) Transforming information, education and communication in Vietnam, Health Education, 103(6): 363–9.

Laverack, G. and Labonte, R. (2000) A planning framework for the accommodation of community empowerment goals within health promotion programming, *Health Policy and Planning*, 15 (3): 255–62.

Laverack, G. and Wallerstein, N. (2001) Measuring community empowerment: a fresh look at organizational domains, *Health Promotion International*, 16(2): 179–85.

Lerner, M. (1986) *Surplus Powerlessness*. Oakland, CA: The Institute for Labour and Mental Health.

Lewaravu, A.K. (1986) *A Training of Trainers in Non-formal, Adult and Community Education in Fiji*. Glasgow: University of Glasgow.

Linney, B. (1995) *Pictures, People and Power. People-centred Visual Aids for Development*. London: Macmillan.

Litwin, M.S. (1995) *How to Measure Survey Reliability and Validity*. London: Sage.

Lloyd, M. and Bor, R. (2004) *Communication Skills for Medicine*, 2nd edn. London: Churchill Livingstone.

London School of Economics (2006) *What is Civil Society?* www.lse.ac.uk/Depts/ ccs/what_is_civil_society.htm, accessed 22 February 2006.

Lupton, B.S., Fonnebo, V., Sogaard, A. J. and Fylkesnes, K. (2005) The Finnmark Intervention Study: do community-based intervention programmes threaten self-rated health and well-being? Experiences from Batsfjord, a fishing village in North Norway, *European Journal of Public Health*, 15(1): 91–6.

Lupton, D. (1995) *The Imperative of Health: Public Health and the Regulated Body*. London: Sage.

MaCallan, L. and Narayan, V. (1994) Keeping the heart beat in Grampian: a case study in community participation and ownership, *Health Promotion International*, 9(1): 13–19.

Manandhar, D.S. *et al.* and members of the MIRA Makwanpur Trial Team (2004) Effect of a participatory intervention with women's groups on birth outcomes in Nepal: cluster-randomised controlled trial, *Lancet*, 364: 970–9.

Marmot, M. and Wilkinson, R.G. (eds) (1999) *Social Determinants of Health*. Oxford: Oxford University Press.

Marshall, G. (1998) *A Dictionary of Sociology*. London: Oxford University Press.

Mays, N. and Pope, C. (1995) Observational methods in health care settings, *British Medical Journal*, 311: 182–4.

Ministry of Health and Ministry of Pacific Island Affairs (2004) *Tupu Ola Moui: Pacific Health Chart Book*. Wellington, NZ: Ministry of Health.

Moana, I. (2005) *Diabetes Prevention in Tongan People*, project report 743. Auckland: University of Auckland.

Murray, S.A. and Graham, L.J.C. (1995) Practice-based needs evaluation: use of four methods in a small neighbourhood, *British Medical Journal*, 310: 1443–8.

North York Community Health Promotion Research Unit (NYCHPRU) (1993) *Community Health Responses to Health Inequalities.* Toronto: NYCHPRU.

O'Connor, M. and Parker, E. (1995) *Health Promotion: Principles and Practice in the Australian Context.* St Leonards, NSW: Allen & Unwin.

O'Gorman, F. (1995) Brazilian community development: changes and challenges, in G. Craig and M. Mayo (eds) *Community Empowerment: A Reader in Participation and Development.* London: Zed Books.

Odedina, F.T., Leader, A.G., Venkataraman, K., Cole, R. and Storm, A. (2000) Feasibility of a community asthma management network (CAMN) program: lessons learnt from an exploratory investigation, *Journal of Social & Administrative Pharmacy*, 17(1): 15–21.

Onyx, J. and Benton, P. (1995) Empowerment and ageing: toward honoured places for crones and sages, in G. Craig and M. Mayo (eds) *Community Empowerment: A Reader in Participation and Development.* London: Zed Books.

Palmer, C.T. and Anderson, M.J. (1986) Assessing the development of community involvement, *World Health Statistics Quarterly*, 39: 345–52.

Patton, M.Q. (1997) Toward distinguishing empowerment evaluation and placing it in a larger context, *Evaluation Practice*, 18(2): 147–63.

Peart, A. and Szoeke, C. (1998) Recreational water use in remote indigenous communities, unpublished report. Canberra: Cooperative Research Centre for Water Quality and Treatment.

Petersen, A.R. (1994) Community development in health promotion: empowerment or regulation? *Australian Journal of Public Health*, 18(2): 213–17.

Photovoice (2006) *Photovoice: Social Change through Photography*, www.photovoice. com accessed 22 August 2006.

Piven, F.F. and Cloward, R. (1977) *Poor Peoples' Movements: Why they Succeed, How they Fail.* New York: Pantheon Books.

Plested, B., Edwards, R. and Jumper-Thurman, P. (2003) *Community Readiness: The Key to Successful Change.* Fort Collins, CO: Tri-ethnic Center for Prevention Research.

Pokhrel, S. and Sauerborn, R. (2004) Household decision-making on child health care in developing countries: the case of Nepal, *Health Policy and Planning*, 19(4): 218–33.

Rappaport, J. (1985) The power of empowerment language, *Social Policy*, autumn: 15–21.

Raven, B.H. and Litman-Adizes, T. (1986) Interpersonal influence and social power in health promotion, in W.B. Ward (ed.) *Advances in Health Education and Promotion.* London: Elsevier.

Rebien, C.C. (1996) Participatory evaluation of development assistance: dealing with power and facilitative learning, *Evaluation*, 2(2): 151–71.

Rifkin, S. (1990) *Community Participation in Maternal and Child Health/Family Planning Programmes.* Geneva: WHO.

Rifkin, S. (2003) A framework linking community empowerment and health equity: it is a matter of CHOICE, *Journal of Health and Population Nutrition*, 21(3): 173.

Rifkin, S. and Pridmore, P. (2001) *Partners in Planning: Information, Participation and Empowerment*. London: MacMillan Education.

Rifkin, S., Muller, F. and Bichmann, W. (1988) Primary health care: on measuring participation, *Social Science & Medicine*, 9: 931–40.

Rissel, C. (1994) Empowerment: the holy grail of health promotion? *Health Promotion International*, 9(1): 39–47.

Rissel, C., Perry, C. and Finnegan, J. (1996) Toward the assessment of psychological empowerment in health promotion: initial tests of validity and reliability, *Journal of the Royal Society of Health*, 116(4): 211–18.

Robertson, A. and Minkler, M. (1994) New health promotion movement: a critical examination, *Health Education Quarterly*, 21(3): 295–12.

Robson, C. (1993) *Real World Research*. Oxford: Blackwell.

Rosengren, A., Wilhelmsen, L. and Orth-Gomer, K. (2004) Coronary disease in relation to social support and social class in Swedish men, *European Heart Journal*, 25(1): 56–63.

Roughan, J.J. (1986) Village organization for development, Ph.D. thesis, Department of Political Science, University of Hawaii.

Rudner-Lugo, N. (1996) Empowerment education. a case study of the resource Sisters/Companeras Program, *Health Education Quarterly*, 23(3): 281–9.

Russell, C.A., Banker Jr, L.J. and Bowman, H.M. (1979) Out-inventing the terrorist, in J. Alexander, D. Carlton and P. Wilkinson (eds) *Terrorism: Theory and Practice*. Boulder, CO: Westview Press.

Russon, C. (1995) The influence of culture on evaluation, *Evaluation Journal of Australasia*, 7(1): 44–9.

Scrimgeour, D. (1997) *Community Control of Aboriginal Health Services in the Northern Territory*. Darwin: Menzies School of Health Research.

Shrestha, S. (2003) A conceptual model for empowerment of the female health volunteers in Nepal, *Education for Health*, 16(3): 318–27.

Shrimpton, R. (1995) Community participation in food and nutrition programmes: an analysis of recent governmental experiences, in P. Pinstrup-Andersen, D. Pellitier and H. Alderman (eds) (1995) *Child Growth and Nutrition in Developing Countries: Priorities for Action*. Ithaca, NY: Cornell University Press.

SLLP (Sustainable Livelihoods for Livestock Producing Communities Project) (2004) *Monitoring and Evaluation Report for December: Sustainable Livelihoods for Livestock Producing Communities*. Bishkek: SLLP.

Smithies, J. and Webster, G. (1998) *Community Involvement in Health*. Aldershot: Ashgate.

Soul City 4 (2001) *Impact Evaluation: Violence Against Women*, vol. 2. Johannesburg: The Institute for Health and Development Communication.

Speer, P. and Hughley, J. (1995) Community organizing: an ecological route to empowerment and power, *American Journal of Community Psychology*, 23(5): 729–48.

Srinivasan, L. (1993) *Tools for Community Participation: A Manual for Training Trainers in Participatory Techniques*. New York: PROWWESS/UNDP.

Starhawk, M.S. (1990) *Truth or Dare? Encounters with Power, Authority and Mystery*. New York: HarperCollins.

Strong, G. (1998) The gentle art of defeating a giant, *The Age*, 21 November 1998: 10.

Syme, L. (1997) Individual vs community interventions in public health practice: some thoughts about a new approach, *Vichealth*, July(2): 2–9.

Taylor, V. (1995) Social reconstruction and community development in the transition to democracy in South Africa, in G. Craig and M. Mayo (eds) *Community Empowerment: A Reader in Participation and Development*. London: Zed Books.

Thomas, P. (2001) Empowering community health: women in Samoa, in D. Pencheorn, C. Guest, D. Melzer and J.A. Muir Gray (eds) *Oxford Handbook of Public Health Practice*. Oxford: Oxford University Press.

Thomson, H., Petticrew, M. and Morrison, D. (2001) Health effects of housing improvement: systematic review of intervention studies, *British Medical Journal*, 323: 187–90.

Thompson, R.J. (1990) Evaluators as change agents: the case of a foreign assistance project in Morocco, *Evaluation and Program Planning*, 13: 379–88.

Tones, K., Tilford, S. and Robinson, Y. (1990) *Health Education: Effectiveness and Efficiency*. London: Chapman & Hall.

Toronto Department of Public Health (1991) *Advocacy for Basic Health Prerequisites: Policy Report*. Toronto: City of Toronto Department of Public Health.

Turbyne, J. (1996) The enigma of empowerment: a study of the transformation of concepts in policy-making processes, Ph.D. thesis, University of Bath.

Turner, B.S. and Samson, C. (1995) *Medical Power and Social Knowledge*. London: Sage.

UNICEF (1977) *Community Involvement in Primary Health Care: A Study of the Process of Community Motivation and Continued Participation*. New York: UNICEF.

Uphoff, N. (1991) A field methodology for participatory self-education, *Community Development Journal*, 26(4): 271–85.

Usher, C.L. (1995) Improving evaluability through self-evaluation, *Evaluation Practice*, 16(1): 59–68.

Wadsworth, Y. and McGuiness, M. (1992) *Understanding Anytime: A Consumer Evaluation of Acute Psychiatric Hospitals*. Melbourne: Mental Illness Awareness Council, VMIAC.

Wagenaar, A., Murray, D. and Toomey, T. (2000) Communities mobilizing for change on alcohol (CMCA): effects of a randomized trial on arrests and traffic crashes, *Addiction*, 95: 209–17.

Wallerstein, N. (1992) Powerlessness, empowerment and health: implications for health promotion programs, *American Journal of Health Promotion,* 6(3): 197–205.

Wallerstein, N. (1998) Identifying and defining the dimensions of community capacity to provide a basis for measurement, *Health Education & Behavior,* 25(3): 258–78.

Wallerstein, N. (2006) *What is the Evidence on Effectiveness of Empowerment to Improve Health?* Copenhagen: WHO Regional Office for Europe.

Wang, C., and Pies, C.A. (2004) Family, maternal and child health through Photovoice, *Maternal and Child Health Journal,* 8(2): 95–102.

Wang, C. Yi, W.K., Tao, Z.W. and Carvano, K. (1998) Photovoice as a participatory health promotion strategy, *Health Promotion International,* 13(1): 75–86.

Wartenberg, T.E. (1990) *The Forms of Power: From Domination to Transformation.* Philadelphia, PA: Temple University Press.

Whitelaw, S., Baxendale, A., Bryce, C., MacHardy, L., Young, I. and Witney, E. (2001) Settings-based health promotion: a review, *Health Promotion International,* 16(4): 339–53.

WHO (World Health Organization) (1986) *Ottawa Charter for Health Promotion.* Geneva: WHO.

WHO (World Health Organization) (1998) *Health Promotion Glossary.* Geneva: WHO.

WHO (World Health Organization) (2001) *Basic Documents,* 43rd edn. Geneva: WHO.

WHO (World Health Organization) (2005) *The Bangkok Charter for Health Promotion in a Globalized World. 6th Global Conference on Health Promotion.* Bangkok: WHO.

WHO (World Health Organization) (2006) *The Definition of Health.* Geneva: WHO.

Wilkinson, R.G. (1996) *Unhealthy Societies: The Afflictions of Inequality.* New York: Routledge.

Wilkinson, R.G. (ed.) (2003) *Social Determinants of Health: The Solid Facts,* 2nd edn. Copenhagen: WHO Regional Office for Europe.

Willis, J. (1987) When is a house not a house? Aspects of the social and physical environment, in SAHC, *Report of Uwankara Palyanyku Kanyuntjaku.* Darwin: SAHC.

Wissmann, J.L. and Tankel, K. (2001) Nursing students' use of a psychopharmacology game for client empowerment, *Journal of Professional Nursing,* 17(2): 101–6.

Zakus, J.D.L. and Lysack, C.L. (1998) Revisiting community participation, *Health Policy and Planning,* 13(1): 1–12.

Zimmerman, M.A. and Rappaport, J. (1988) Citizen participation, perceived control and psychological empowerment, *American Journal of Community Psychology,* 16(5): 725–43.

Index